The Microscopic Colitis Diet Book

Other books by this author

- **Microscopic Colitis**
- **Understanding Microscopic Colitis**
- **Vitamin D and Autoimmune Disease**
- **8 Ways to Prevent Pancreatic Cancer**
- **Why Magnesium Is the Key to Long-Term Health**
- **Stroke Recovery**

The Microscopic Colitis Diet Book

Choosing a Safe Diet for Microscopic Colitis Patients

Wayne Persky

Persky Farms

United States

First published and distributed in the United States of America by:

Persky Farms, 19242 Darrs Creek Rd, Bartlett, TX 76511-4460. Tel.: (1)254-718-1125; Fax: (1)254-527-3682. www.perskyfarms.com

ISBN 978-1-7364066-9-4

Contents

Chapter 1

Why it's necessary to change our diet.

Probably the earliest attempts to use diet changes to treat microscopic colitis (MC), or any other inflammatory bowel disease (IBD) was done by using the specific carbohydrate diet (SCD), which was promoted by Elaine Gottschall. Gottschall had a daughter who had ulcerative colitis, and who was a patient of Dr. Sidney V Haas.

Haas had described the first SCD in 1924, to use in the treatment of children who had celiac disease. The diet was also known as the banana diet, because in a medical trial of 10 children, all eight of those treated with bananas went into remission, and the other two, who were controls, died.

Celiac disease had typically caused a mortality rate of about one in four children (who had celiac disease), before the banana diet was discovered. In 1951, Haas published a medical textbook called *The Management of Celiac Disease*, that described the SCD as a treatment for not only celiac disease, but also, IBD.

Regrettably, when wheat was discovered to be the actual cause of celiac disease, during World War II, Haas never accepted that fact. Instead, he continued to insist that the problem was starch, and denied that wheat gluten was the cause of celiac disease.

Elaine Gottschall was a biochemist who began to promote the SCD in 1996, when she published her book, *Breaking the Vicious Cycle*. In the book, she described how her daughter had been cured of ulcerative colitis in two years by following the SCD, and she suggested that the diet she described could cure various medical conditions, although she didn't provide any supporting data. Not only did she promote the SCD as a treatment for Crohn's disease, ulcerative colitis, and celiac disease, but she also stated that it could be used to treat chronic diarrhea, diverticulitis, cystic fibrosis, and even autism. In retrospect, those claims appear to have been a bit overly ambitious, although more than a few patients who had various diseases, were probably able to gain remission by using the SCD she recommended. Unfortunately, although the SCD may bring remission for some MC patients, most of us cannot tolerate certain foods that are allowed by the SCD, so we will continue to react if we follow that diet.

What about the other diets that some patients have tried to use to treat MC?

Over the years, some MC patients have been able to reach remission by using a diet developed for some other purpose. Examples of this are the paleo diet, the autoimmune protocol (AIP) diet, and the fermentable oligosaccharides, disaccharides, monosaccharides, and polyols (FODMAP) diet, for example, in addition to the specific carbohydrate diet (SCD). But while these diets sometimes work to successfully bring remission for some

Why it's necessary to change our diet.

MC patients, none of them can be used to bring remission for most of us, unless certain specifications in their rules are changed. They all contain basic flaws that prevent them from being capable of successfully bringing (and maintaining) remission for the vast majority of MC patients.

A diet used to control the symptoms of MC should be effective for most of us, not just some of us. Accordingly, an effective microscopic colitis diet uses some of the recommendations from all of these diets, while avoiding those diet recommendations that are contraindicated for MC patients.

Many gastroenterologists still deny that MC can be controlled by diet changes.

But of course, out in the real world, many thousands of MC patients have been able to successfully reach remission, and remain there, simply by removing certain foods from their diet. These are foods that cause our immune systems to produce antibodies against them.

Although we may choose to fine-tune our long-term diet from time to time, after we reach remission, our initial recovery, for each and every one of us, can usually be based on a simple elimination diet, that totally avoids certain foods that cause most MC patients to react. The term "totally" is crucial to the success of the diet, because if we allow even very small traces of certain foods to sneak into our diet, we may not be able to successfully reach remission, because the inflammation will continue at a level sufficient to perpetuate the disease.

Most of us are not born with food sensitivities.

So why would diet changes help to control MC? The answer to this question can be found by examining the damage to our intestines that can result from prolonged (chronic) inflammation.

Normally, when food is digested, it's broken down very thoroughly into individual amino acids and very short amino acid chains. These nutrients are then absorbed through the mucosal lining of our small intestine, into our bloodstream, and then they are carried to cells throughout the body, wherever they are needed. The surface of the mucosal lining of our small intestine contains perpendicularly-oriented, elongated cells, known as enterocytes, and the spaces between the enterocytes are known as tight junctions. Normally, these tight junctions open just enough to allow the individual amino acids and very short amino acid chains to pass through into our bloodstream.

Chronic intestinal inflammation causes leaky gut.

MC develops as a result of chronic inflammation due to certain health issues that cause compromised digestion for an extended period. These health issues can be the result of using certain medications, parasites, bacterial infections, or even experiencing extreme stress, especially chronic stress (long-term stress). Regardless of the initial cause of compromised digestion, as a result, certain foods may be only partially digested. This can result in many partially digested, medium length amino acid chains. And unfortunately, published research shows that when the intestines are inflamed, the tight junctions tend to open much wider than normal. This is known in medical circles as increased intestinal permeability, and it's referred to by others as leaky gut. When leaky gut occurs, some of the medium length chains of amino acids that can result from partially digested food, are able to pass through the tight junctions into the bloodstream.

Leaky gut causes food sensitivities.

The immune system immediately detects these longer chains, because obviously, they shouldn't be in the bloodstream, and it flags them as foreign invaders, or pathogens. Our adaptive immune system will then initiate an allergic reaction against them. Consequently, in the future, whenever those particular amino acid chains, (peptides) show up in the bloodstream, the production of antibodies against them will be triggered. And those antibodies will alert macrophages and other white cells designed to destroy pathogens, so that they will go after the invaders. That means that in the future, the food from which those reactive amino acid chains were cleaved, will trigger an immune reaction whenever it is eaten. Note that foods that are capable of becoming sensitivity issues are always proteins (except for one specific exception, which will be discussed later).

No one can digest gluten.

Because humans evolved during the paleolithic period of history, before wheat was developed, the human digestive system is incapable of fully digesting wheat — no one can properly (completely) digest wheat. Wheat was developed during the neolithic period, only about 10,000 years ago. The main problem with wheat is the primary protein, gluten. Because of our inability to digest gluten completely, whenever we eat wheat, relatively large amounts of reactive amino acid chains remain undigested. This is true for everyone, not just MC patients. For most people, however, these partially digested elements simply pass on through their digestive system, and out the other end of their digestive tract, without creating any significant problems.

For celiacs, unfortunately, their genetic heritage allows these partially-digested amino acid sequences to pass through the tight junctions of their small intestine, to contaminate their bloodstream, and thereby trigger a typical celiac reaction. MC patients have a similar problem due to the fact that the inflammation that causes the disease, also causes leaky gut, which allows the partially digested amino acid sequences to pass through the tight junctions in the lining of their intestines to similarly contaminate their bloodstream. Medical research exists to show that gluten can cause a leaky gut problem where it did not previously exist (Hollon, et al., 2015).[1]

Virtually all MC patients are sensitive to gluten.

Because of the unique feature described in the last sentence of the paragraph above, virtually all MC patients are sensitive to gluten. Those few who can demonstrate that they do not react to gluten, have developed a tolerance for it, despite the fact that their immune system produces antibodies to it, similar to the way many celiacs are asymptomatic, despite being sensitive to gluten. There doesn't appear to be any medical research to verify this, but presumably, asymptomatic celiacs are subject to the same increased risk of developing non-Hodgkin's lymphoma, as untreated symptomatic celiacs. And if that's true, it should follow that MC patients who are asymptomatic to gluten exposure, are also subject to a similar increased risk.

MC is commonly associated with certain food sensitivities.

Certain foods are much more likely to produce an immune system reaction than others, and as we shall see later, those foods tend to be proteins. And as mentioned above, the most serious food sensitivity for MC patients, by far, is gluten.

In general, the preceding pages describe how food sensitivities associated with MC are developed. And so this is why avoiding those specific inflammatory foods is an effective way to control this disease. Many gastroenterologists are still unwilling to admit that these food sensitivities are specifically the source of the chronic inflammation that perpetuates the symptoms of MC. While some gastroenterologists may understand how food sensitivities are created, apparently, many of them consider this to be the domain of allergists, and therefore, outside their specialty.

For many of us, the medical approach simply does not work.

The medical approach to treating MC involves attempting to suppress the inflammation in the intestines that appears to cause the disease. However, note that the official medical treatment typically involves no attempt to prevent the inflammation from developing in the first place. Without diet changes to avoid the inflammatory foods, the medical treatment merely attempts to suppress the inflammation after it develops.

It usually doesn't take long for most MC patients to realize that the typical medical treatment, consisting of the prescription of inflammation suppressing drugs, will only provide temporary relief, provided that it is even effective at all for them. For some patients, the medications that are prescribed never bring relief — not even temporarily.

Budesonide is usually prescribed as the first line of treatment.

The most popular medical treatment prescribed to treat MC is budesonide, and published medical research shows that over 80% of patients who are able to get relief using budesonide, relapse after the treatment is ended. Most gastroenterologists are reluctant to prescribe budesonide for more than a few months. Often, many of them seem to be willing to renew the prescription a few times, especially if the dosage is reduced. But in some cases, this will only occur if the prescription renewal is requested by the patient.

Doctors are trained to write prescriptions for drugs, not diets.

In medical school, medical students receive very limited training regarding nutrition and diet issues. Doctors are trained to treat disease by writing prescriptions for powerful drugs that have been approved by the Food and Drug Administration (FDA) for the treatment of specific disease. Unfortunately, there are no FDA approved drugs specifically labeled for treating MC, so whenever a doctor writes a prescription for the treatment of MC, it will be for an off label use of a drug approved for the treatment of Crohn's disease or ulcerative colitis. But the main point here is that it's not surprising that doctors would have a problem understanding food sensitivities, considering that they receive such a small amount of training on identifying and treating food sensitivity issues while they're in medical school

Gastroenterologists have been generally reluctant to embrace diet as a legitimate treatment.

Gastroenterologists have traditionally insisted that MC cannot be controlled by diet changes simply because researchers have never published a double-blind, random study demonstrating compelling evidence that diet can be used to successfully control the disease. Of course, no one has ever published a study showing that diet changes cannot be used to treat MC, either, but doctors always assume that if a treatment hasn't been officially proven, over and over again, to be effective, based on published studies, then it must not be effective. But if we examine this situation more closely, we can easily see why this problem exists..

Most medical trials are funded by the big pharmaceutical companies.

They use the trials to prove the efficacy of certain drugs that they have developed, in order to satisfy the requirements of the FDA. Before the FDA will consider granting an approval for any drug, the manufacturer must prove that that drug is at least significantly more effective than a placebo, for treating the disease for which the drug is to be labeled, and the drug must be shown to be generally safe for that specific use.

The Microscopic Colitis Diet Book

It costs hundreds of thousands of dollars, to conduct a clinical trial these days, so it's certainly not difficult to understand why any drug company would not be interested in financing a study to show that a disease can be treated without the use of any medications. And the increasing costs of these studies is just one of several reasons why drugs developed today are ridiculously expensive and out of reach for many patients unless they have insurance assistance.

Of course some studies are conducted by universities or other institutions with government, or industry funding. But the studies selected to be funded by such grants definitely do not involve a process, or a type of treatment that has been claimed to be ineffective by the medical profession. And a study that would conclusively prove the effectiveness of diet changes for the treatment of MC, would be extremely expensive because there are so many foods that would have to be considered in a study of this type. Medical trials typically consider only one, or a comparison of two or three treatments, in order to simplify the management, and keep the total cost of the trial within reasonable limits. So the odds of any prestigious research organization agreeing to undertake a study designed to prove that MC can be effectively controlled by diet changes is about as likely as winning the lottery.

Therefore, most gastronterologists can't offer MC patients an optional treatment based on diet changes, simply because their official departmental policies do not include an officially accepted policy that allows treatment by diet. That said, a relatively small percentage of gastroenterologists are beginning to recognize that even though they don't have an official policy regarding diet. when treating microscopic colitis patients, as individuals, they have begun to recognize that certain foods, especially gluten and dairy products, do indeed have a significant effect on when trying to control the disease.

Perhaps the most important reason for using diet changes to control MC is to avoid having to use powerful drugs.

As previously mentioned, there are no drugs labeled for treating microscopic colitis, so all medications used to treat this disease are prescribed for off label use. A couple of decades ago, the only medications that were commonly prescribed to treat MC were prednisone, sulfasalazine, mesalamine, bismuth subsalicylate, colestyramine, antidiarrheals, and immunosuppressants.

Steroids have always been the treatment of choice for MC. But Prednisone and most earlier steroids were notorious for their draconian side effects. When budesonide was approved for treating IBD's, it quickly became the primary prescribed treatment for MC (despite the fact that it wasn't labeled for MC). Because budesonide is not activated until it reaches the terminal ilium, and the colon, it greatly reduces the systemic side effect issues so common with most steroids. In many cases, if the budesonide treatment fails, or a patient relapses after a treatment is ended, an immunosuppressant is prescribed. Most immune system suppressants are either chemotherapy drugs that were originally designed for organ transplant patients, or they are tumor necrosis factor (TNF) blockers. Consequently, most drugs prescribed to treat MC carry risks for producing some very undesirable side effects for many patients.

Today, many doctors are prescribing biologicals.

Biologicals comprise a unique class of drugs. While conventional drugs are formulated from synthetic chemicals by using ordinary laboratory techniques, biologicals, (or biologics), are produced by using live cells from animals, plants, or micro-organisms to generate monoclonal antibodies (MAbs) that tend to bind to a specific pro-inflammatory protein, thereby deactivating it. The production of biologics tends to be complex and widely varying, but a common thread is the fact that the first step in the production of a biologic typically involves genetic engineering.

In 1982, when the first genetically modified organism (GMO) product was approved by the FDA, the concept was typically met with nothing but wrath from the public. Although four decades have gone by since then, many people still avoid products that contain GMOs, whenever possible. Consequently, these days, industries involved with the development and use of GMO products rarely (if ever) mention the term (GMO). Instead, they describe the technology they are using with quite different language that is difficult for most individuals to interpret, and therefore they are less likely to associate the product with GMO technology. Are patients who are using biologicals to treat their health issues these days even aware that they are allowing the infusion of a product developed by genetic engineering techniques into their bloodstream, or allowing it to be injected into one of their muscles?

Controlling MC by using diet changes is natural and safe.

By comparison, the diet changes needed to control MC are relatively economical, and they are a totally natural process, so they have absolutely none of the side effect risks imposed by medical treatments. And unlike using medications, using diet changes to control a disease will not become less effective, or totally ineffective, as the years go by — using diet changes to control the disease will continue to work as long as the proper diet changes are maintained. By contrast, medications tend to lose effectiveness as time goes by, because the body learns to adjust for their use, and eventually, most medications will progressively lose some of their effectiveness, and some will eventually fail to provide any benefits at all.

The microscopic colitis diet is a set of guidelines for selecting safe foods for MC patients, rather than being just a list of foods.

Because of the way MC affects us, although we all have certain similar characteristics, with regard to symptoms, we're all different, and we have different food sensitivities. Therefore, the microscopic colitis diet is not as much a specific list of acceptable, and unacceptable foods, as a list of rules that will allow anyone to determine their particular food sensitivities, and select a recovery diet, accordingly. By following these guidelines, most MC patients should be able to reach remission, and stay in remission, without a need for any medications.

Alternatively, those patients who wish to use diet changes to help their medical treatment work more effectively, or those who want to use the diet so that they can wean off a medical treatment, will find that the microscopic colitis diet works well for that purpose, also.

Nothing provides perfect control for MC, not even the MC diet.

Although using diet changes to control MC works well for most of us, realistically, under real world conditions, we have to acknowledge the fact that nothing works for everyone. Experience shows that a very small percentage, possibly about three or four percent of MC patients who attempt to control their symptoms by changing their diet, are, for whatever reason, unsuccessful. Usually, when that happens, it's because an inflammatory item in the diet is being overlooked, or something in the diet is somehow cross contaminated. But regardless of the cause, a few people have problems achieving complete remission by making diet changes, without the use of any medications.

But this situation commonly occurs with every known treatment for every disease. It happens very frequently with medical treatments. For example, whenever Doctors write a prescription, although they typically give their patients the impression that a drug they are prescribing will resolve the patient's symptoms, the reality is that many drugs are actually only marginally more effective than a placebo. A few of the most effective drugs will provide benefits for about two-thirds to maybe three-fourths of the patients to whom they are prescribed, but this is not common. Most medications are far less effective. In the case of biologicals, for example, one published medical study that analyzed treatment trials of Crohn's patients for several of the most popular biologicals, showed very disappointing results. When they considered the total number of people who participated in the trials, they found that the final net clinical remission rates at the end of the follow-up period were approximately 17% for Remicade, 29% for Humira, 19% for Entyvio, and 14% for Stelara (Long, 2022, March 16).[2]

But even in the few cases where the MC diet does not bring remission, there is a solution.

Fortunately, in almost every case where the proper diet changes alone will not bring relief, budesonide can be used in conjunction with the diet, to bring remission, and as the intestines heal, the budesonide dose can be tapered to a very small maintenance dose that will provide the extra boost needed to maintain remission.

Published medical research is available to verify that long-term use of budesonide at relatively low doses is safe (Münch, et al., 2016).[3] So there is a way for virtually anyone and everyone to use diet changes to successfully control their MC symptoms, even if they should need a small maintenance dose of an anti-inflammatory medication in order to maintain remission.

No substantial medical dietary data are available.

Please note that as of this date, at least, no significant medical research studies have been published regarding dietary treatment of microscopic colitis. Consequently, the information in this

The Microscopic Colitis Diet Book

book is based on epidemiological data taken from the shared experiences of thousands of microscopic colitis patients who live with the disease, and who have generously shared their experiences in posts to the Microscopic Colitis Discussion and Support Board located at the following Internet address:

https://www.perskyfarms.com/phpBB/index.php

This is the longest-running microscopic colitis discussion forum on the Internet, and as of this date, it has been in continuous operation for over 17 years, and it contains the largest database in the world of actual experiences shared by microscopic colitis patients.

Summary

Medical treatments for microscopic colitis are not always successful, and even when they are, they provide only temporary relief. In order to obtain long-term relief, certain diet changes must be made. Although many different diets have been used by microscopic colitis patients, in order to reach remission, none of them have been found to work effectively for all MC patients. They all require certain modifications in order to meet the personal needs of most individual microscopic colitis patients.

Chapter 2

Discovering our food sensitivities.

It's important to note that we must track down and avoid all of our food sensitivities, not just some, or most of them. If we over-look a food that's causing our immune system to produce anti-bodies, continuing to eat that food will probably prevent us from reaching remission, despite eliminating all of our other food sensitivities from our diet. Basically, there are two ways to deter-mine which foods must be eliminated from our diet in order to stop the inflammation that perpetuates the reactions that cause the persistent symptoms of this disease.

1. Adopt an elimination diet.
2. Select foods based on EnteroLab stool test results.

Using an elimination diet to reach remission.

The elimination diet works to bring remission by eliminating **all** of the foods that are known to typically be inflammatory for most MC patients. This is a shotgun approach, and it typically excludes a few foods that many MC patients can tolerate. But since all food sensitivities for any particular MC patient is unknown early on in most patients' recovery programs, it's necessary for anyone who chooses to use an elimination diet to avoid these foods, because they are definitely a problem for most of us. As mentioned previously, if one or more of these foods happen to be a problem for someone who is attempting to use an elimination diet, and they do not eliminate that food, or those foods from their diet, they will probably not be able to reach remission.

Gluten absolutely must be eliminated from a recovery diet.

An elimination diet must exclude all possible sources of gluten, which means all derivatives of wheat, rye, or barley. Even trace amounts as small as those in medications and supplements must be avoided. Some skincare products and shampoos contain gluten, and should be avoided. Even the glue on envelopes may contain gluten, and if it does, and you lick it, you will react a few hours later. Read the labels carefully, on anything, and everything you use, especially anything that will go into your mouth.

Casein must also be eliminated from our diet.

Likewise, avoid all products that contain any derivatives of casein, the primary protein in milk. This means that you must avoid all dairy products, because all dairy products contain casein. Even some so-called "nondairy creamers" contain casein, so they must be avoided. The manufacturers of these products mistakenly assume that most people who are dairy intolerant, are lactose intolerant, not casein. intolerant.

While it's true that anyone whose intestines are inflamed is lactose intolerant, this is pretty much a moot point for MC patients, because casein is a much bigger problem than lactose. True, we are lactose intolerant whenever we are reacting, but lactose intolerance only causes poor digestion. The partially digested lactose passes into our colon, where it's fermented by opportunistic gut bacteria, resulting in gas, bloating, cramps, and diarrhea. But lactose does not trigger the production of anti-bodies, so while it's a temporary cause of diarrhea, it does not trigger MC reactions the way that true food sensitivities do.

Note that all products derived from any type of milk contain casein.

Casein is the primary protein in milk. More than one type of casein exists, however. A1 β-casein is found in the milk of most dairy cows in the herds on dairy farms these days, while some less common types of dairy cows produce milk containing a high percentage of A2 β-casein. A2 β-casein has been shown to be far less inflammatory for most people than A1 β-casein.

Although the milk from certain types of cows, or goats containing high percentages of A2 β-casein has been shown to be easier to digest, and less inflammatory for people in the general population, this is a moot point for MC patients, because even minuscule amounts of A1 β-casein will trigger a reaction for those of us who are sensitive to casein. The milk from all types of domestic cows, and all goats contains at least a small percentage of A1 β-casein, so therefore, milk from all cows and goats must be avoided, without exception

Milk from camelids is a safe exception.

Camelids include camels, llamas, alpacas, vicuñas and guanacos, and the milk from these animals is generally safe for us, because it contains a different type of casein. Again, this is a moot point for most MC patients, because it's very unlikely that most people, in most parts of the world, would have access to milk from any of these animals. That said, a few camel dairies do exist, so camelid milk is available in some locations, for individuals who feel that they absolutely must have a source of safe milk.

Alpha gal is the only sugar known to cause the production of antibodies.

Lactose is a sugar, and our immune system only produces antibodies against certain proteins. That said, there is one exception to this rule, known as alpha gal allergy. Alpha gal is short for galactose-alpha-1,3-galactose, which is a sugar. Most mammals contain the sugar in the cells of their body. Even the so-called tenderizing solutions containing natural flavorings that are often injected into poultry, may contain alpha gal. Alpha gal allergy is also known as mammalian meat allergy.

It's believed that this allergy is spread by the bite of the Lone Star tick. Although it's still somewhat rare, it's spreading in many parts of the world. If a person has mammalian meat allergy, they become ill after eating the meat from any mammal, or as mentioned above, certain poultry that have been injected with certain natural flavoring, so they have to avoid these meats. Aside from that uncommon issue, as mentioned above, we're only sensitive to certain proteins.

Soy, and legumes, must be avoided with an elimination diet.

This requires careful attention, because derivatives of soy are found in many products at the supermarket. Most of the gums used as thickeners in many liquids are derived from legumes, and many of us are sensitive to gums made by other processes, as well. Beans, peas, and peanuts are legumes, of course, so the requirement to avoid them eliminates most plant-based sources of protein. Soy derivatives are used as emulsifiers in many products, and soy oil is widely used.

Note that soy oil is a problem for many of us.

Most experts agree that soy oil should not be a problem for people who are sensitive to soy. But the experts are wrong — many of us do indeed react to soy oil. The issue here is that oil refining processes are never perfect. Consequently, soy oil commonly contains a tiny fraction of one percent of soya protein, and this tiny amount is enough to cause some of us to react.

Eggs should be avoided.

About two thirds of us are sensitive to chicken eggs, so eggs should be avoided while on the elimination diet. After remission is achieved, some of us can tolerate other types of eggs, such as duck eggs, especially if we use them only in baked goods, rather than as whole fried, scrambled, or hard-boiled eggs. Duck eggs are sometimes available at supermarkets and farmers markets. But, of course, like any other food, they should be tested, before being added to the diet, after reaching remission.

A food and reaction journal can be very helpful.

While recovering, it can be very helpful to keep a journal where every food eaten, and how we feel, for up to a day afterward, are recorded. This information can be reviewed from time to time in order to detect problems with the current diet. The contents of each meal, and snack should be recorded, including any supplements or medications that are being used.

Any item that goes into our mouth, or onto our skin, should be noted in the journal. When reviewing the information, we have to be aware that food allergies will cause a reaction within seconds or minutes, whereas food sensitivities will cause reactions within a few hours to a day or more later.

What's the difference between a food allergy and a food sensitivity?

A classic food allergy causes an immunoglobulin E (IgE)-based reaction that normally begins to become apparent from a few minutes to 15 or 20 minutes after beginning to eat an item. But in some cases, especially with anaphylactic type reactions, a reaction can begin within a few seconds of beginning to eat. An (IgE)-based reaction can result in redness of affected areas on the skin, swelling, itching, or pain, such as the reaction that is seen from a mosquito bite, or a wasp's sting. This type of immune system reaction causes the degranulation of mast cells in the area of the bite or sting, which releases histamine and other pro-inflammatory mediators. The redness and swelling is promoted by the histamine and other inflammatory mediators.

A serious allergy may result in anaphylaxis.

If a patient is truly allergic to a food, sting, or insect bite, the IgE-based reaction may escalate immediately to anaphylactic symptoms. The patient may go into shock, with a sudden drop in blood pressure, a constriction of the airways that typically causes breathing difficulty, tachycardia (rapid heartbeat), a weak pulse, and possibly heart palpitations. There will usually be a rash on the chest or face, and there may be nausea and vomiting. Obviously, a reaction of this seriousness may be life-threatening.

MC causes food sensitivities, rather than food allergies.

The immune system reactions caused by food sensitivities proceed very differently from food allergies. Typically, they begin 3 to 6 hours after a food is eaten. This is because normally, those foods will have passed through the stomach, and into the small intestine, before a reaction is triggered. Reactions of this type are based on immunoglobulin A (IgA) reactions, and although the mucosal lining of the intestines contain a relatively high density of IgA receptors, IgA receptors can be found in all mucosal linings, meaning that IgA responses can also be triggered in the mouth, or the esophagus, in addition to the intestines, in some cases. Because of this, the response time before an immune system reaction begins can vary by hours. But in most cases, as noted above, IgA reactions typically begin about 3 to 6 hours after a meal is consumed.

A few other foods must be minimized.

When selecting foods for an elimination diet, other factors in addition to immune system reactions must be considered. For example, while our intestines are inflamed, the ability of our small intestine to produce digestive enzymes is compromised. As a result, we slowly lose the ability to produce normal amounts of the enzymes necessary for digesting certain foods, especially carbohydrates. Consequently, we become unable to completely digest normal amounts of these foods. This means that we may be better able to digest smaller meals, or snacks, eaten more often, than the fewer, larger meals that we would otherwise normally eat.

Early on, sugar is a problem.

Sugar is especially hard to digest, and should be minimized in a recovery diet. Artificial sweeteners, especially aspartame, should generally be totally avoided. The only artificial sweetener that has been found to be normally safe for most MC patients who are on a recovery diet, is any sweetener based on the Stevia leaf. Otherwise, it's best to use minimal amounts of ordinary cane sugar, known as sucrose, or small amounts of natural sweeteners such as honey, or maple sugar.

During recovery, fiber is a problem.

Fiber's claim to fame is the ability to supposedly maintain bowel regularity, by reducing constipation. But this tends to make it counterproductive if used to minimize diarrhea. Published medical research shows that random, double-blind trials prove that while fiber may bulk up the stool somewhat to give the illusion of reducing diarrhea, it actually tears the cells in the tissues exposed at the surface of the lining of the colon. Consequently, the body is forced to replace those cells as soon as possible. This has to be done by the immune system, because the immune system is responsible for taking care of all cellular healing required by the body.

Whenever an IBD is active, the immune system already has more than it can handle, so it certainly doesn't need any more intestinal damage that has to be repaired. Because of this, the net result of too much fiber in the diet is increased irritation. While fiber doesn't cause the production of antibodies, it is highly irritating to an already-inflamed colon. Consequently, if we don't minimize our fiber intake during recovery, it may cause enough irritation of our colon to prevent us from being able to reach remission. This means, for example, if rice is selected as part of a recovery diet, white rice should be chosen, rather than brown rice.

Fructose is digested by the liver.

The primary sugar found in most fruits is fructose. Fruits also contain sugar alcohols, such as sorbitol. Sugar alcohols are indigestible. This means that they pass into the colon undigested, where they are often fermented by opportunistic gut bacteria.

The fermentation process typically results in the production of gas, which causes bloating, and sometimes cramps and diarrhea. This can make fruits especially difficult to digest before we reach remission.

Fructose calories are unmonitored.

Additionally, because fructose is digested by the liver, rather than the digestive system, it doesn't trigger the release of insulin, as other sugars do. Consequently, the body has no way of monitoring its satiation level, and so it isn't as capable of knowing when it has had enough (or too much). In other words, it isn't able to keep track of the calorie intake from fructose, the way it does with other sugars. This causes problems for people who are on a calorie restricted diet.

Citric acid is a problem.

We usually can't tolerate more than relatively small amounts of citric acid while we're recovering. Because of that, citrus fruits, and any drink that contains citric acid, should be avoided during recovery. Note that although tomatoes are actually part of the nightshade family of plants, they contain high levels of citric acid, similar to citrus fruits, and so tomatoes, and any products derived from them, should be avoided during recovery.

Foods should be overcooked.

Foods selected for a recovery diet should be overcooked, to make digestion easier. And spices should be generally avoided for a recovery diet. Small amounts of salt are usually safe, but spicy foods should be avoided until after remission has been achieved, and the intestines have at least partially healed.

A recovery diet should be high in protein.

Generally speaking, a recovery diet should be relatively high in protein, because the healing process requires a lot of protein, and healing the intestines, especially, requires a lot of protein, in order to heal all the damage caused by the chronic inflammation.

Summarizing the elimination diet.

Basically, the elimination diet requires avoiding gluten, casein, soy (and legumes), and eggs, and minimizing fiber and sugar. All vegetables should be peeled and over-cooked, and fruits should be minimized. All raw vegetables and fruit, with the exception of bananas, should be avoided in a recovery diet. Iceberg lettuce, especially, should be totally avoided. Citric acid, spices, and all artificial sweeteners, except for sweeteners derived from the leaves of the Stevia plant, should be avoided. A recovery diet should be simple, bland, and consist of as few foods as possible, preferably about 1/2 dozen or less, but certainly no more than eight or 10 basic foods. A recovery diet must not be used to experiment with foods. That should be done after remission is attained.

Using stool testing to achieve remission.

Why would we choose to use the stool tests offered by EnteroLab?

There are many other tests available for detecting food sensitivities. Why can't they be used? The answer to that is, they can be used, of course, but an examination of combined patient experiences shows that virtually all the alternative tests available, have extremely poor accuracy for determining the type of food sensitivities associated with MC. Examples of unsatisfactory tests are tests which are based on blood tests, or skin tests.

Blood tests and skin tests are virtually always designed to detect IgE reactions.

Tests of this type typically show many false positive and false negative results if used to test for food sensitivities. This means that patients who use those tests will be avoiding some foods that they could be safely eating, and they will still be eating some foods that they should be avoiding, because those foods are causing their immune system to produce antibodies against them. Blood tests and skin tests are virtually worthless for detecting the food sensitivities that cause MC.

MC is associated with IgA reactions.

The type of immune system reactions caused by the food sensitivities associated with MC are IgA-based reactions. And these are the reactions that perpetuate the inflammation that causes MC. This type of reaction causes the lymphocytic infiltration into the epithelial cells in the lining of the colon, that's used as a diagnostic marker for the disease.

So the primary reason why the stool tests work so well, while the other types of tests do not, is simply because most other types of tests look for IgE-based antibodies, rather than IgA-based antibodies. IgA antibodies are produced in the colon, and they are rarely found in the blood in concentrations sufficient to allow accurate detection.

These IGA antibodies are concentrated in the colon.

Consequently, even if the tests based on blood samples or skin tests, which are normally used by immunologists, were designed to detect IgA antibodies, they would still be virtually worthless for attempting to determine food sensitivities associated with MC, because these tests look for antibodies in the wrong location, namely the blood, or the skin. The proper place to look for food sensitivity antibodies is the lining of the intestines, or the stool.

Currently, EnteroLab is the only practical choice for determining food sensitivities.

EnteroLab is the only laboratory in the world offering stool tests for detecting food sensitivities that can be purchased by patients anywhere in the world. And after decades of operation, they have an exemplary track record of providing consistently prompt, accurate, and reliable results. Their tests can be ordered by anyone, online, or by phone.

The lab supplies a test kit to simplify collecting the sample, and after the sample is collected, it can be properly packaged (according to the directions), frozen, and shipped back to the laboratory by overnight delivery. The test results are emailed to the patient, along with a doctor's interpretation of the results, as soon as they are available.

Most MC patients will find the combination of test panels A1 + C1 to be the most useful. A direct link to the lab, where those tests are described, can be found at the link below.

https://www.enterolab.com/StaticPages/TestInfo.aspx#PanelA1C1

Patients who are following a vegetarian or vegan diet, will find test panels A 2+ C2 to be the most useful.

EnteroLab's main webpage can be found at the link below:

https://www.enterolab.com/

Here's why the A1 + C1 panels are a good choice.

The A1 and C1 panels of tests utilize standard laboratory ELISA tests designed to detect antibodies to the most common foods that normally cause MC patients to react. These include gluten, casein, soy, chicken eggs, oats, corn, rice, beef, pork, chicken, tuna, almonds, cashews, walnuts, and white potato. Tests for additional foods are not included, because for most MC patients, those additional foods are rarely a problem, and including tests for those foods in the panels would only significantly increase the total cost of the panels for everyone, while providing little, or no benefit.

MC often causes malabsorption of the nutrients in food.

Those who are curious about how much damage the inflammation caused by their food sensitivities has done to their intestines, and their ability to absorb nutrients from their food, can order a fecal fat test. The fecal fat test measures the amount of unabsorbed fat remaining in a stool sample. This result provides a good way to estimate the degree to which our ability to absorb nutrients may be compromised. Malabsorption of nutrients is a common problem for MC patients until they get the disease under control, and their intestines begin to heal.

When ordering a stool test to detect food sensitivities, we should remember that these tests are designed to detect food sensitivities that are currently in our diet. If we have been avoiding a food for more than a few months, antibodies to that food are much more difficult to detect, because antibody levels slowly decay over time, after a food is no longer eaten. Gluten anti-bodies are much more persistent, and gluten sensitivity can be detected even after we have been avoiding all foods that contain gluten, for up to about two years. This is because gluten anti-bodies (antigliadin antibodies) have a half-life of 120 days, whereas antibodies to most foods have a half-life of about five or six days.

Therefore, if we wish to use an EnteroLab test to verify whether or not we are sensitivity to a specific food that we have been avoiding for a relatively long period of time, adding it into our diet about a week or more before we collect the test sample to send to the lab, will ensure that it's properly tested. From a prac-tical viewpoint, however, if we already know that a particular food definitely causes us to react, there would be little point in punishing ourselves by adding it back into our diet. Therefore, we should only do this with foods that we are not sure about, and we want a medical test result to verify our opinion.

Summary

An elimination diet that avoids all of the foods known to cause reactions for most MC patients can be used to bring remission from MC if it's properly followed. Alternatively, if the proper stool tests are ordered from EnteroLab, the offending foods can be identified by the lab, so that they can be eliminated from the diet, which typically makes recovery faster and easier for most MC patients.

Discovering our food sensitivities.

Most MC patients find the A1 +C1 test panels to be the most helpful. Those following a vegan or a vegetarian diet typically find the A2 + C2 test panels to be the most helpful.

Chapter 3

Issues to consider when selecting a recovery diet.

Whether we use an elimination diet, or stool tests from EnteroLab, selecting safe foods for our recovery diet is vital, if we hope to control the symptoms of this disease. The primary difference at this point will be that if we chose to order stool tests from EnteroLab, at least we will be relatively sure which foods we cannot safely eat. And if we don't have any test results, although everyone's individual test results will be slightly different, we can use the test results from a large number of MC patients, to determine a diet that will be safe for most of us.

For example, we know that every one of us reacts to gluten. And we know that about 2/3 to 3/4 of us also react to casein, or soy, or chicken eggs, or some combination of these foods. Therefore, an elimination diet should avoid all of them, in order to minimize the risk of selecting an inflammatory food for our recovery diet.

The reason for eliminating all of them, of course, is that if we continue to eat even a single food that is causing our immune system to produce antibodies, then we will probably never be able to reach remission, regardless of how many other foods we avoid. We have to totally avoid every food that causes our immune system to produce antibodies, not just most of them, in order to get to remission.

That said, if we have recent EnteroLab test results in hand, and those results show that one or more of those foods listed above do not cause us to react, then any foods shown to be safe by the EnteroLab test results can be safely included in a recovery diet. Without EnteroLab test results showing them to be safe, though, we definitely need to avoid all of them in our recovery diet.

Gluten and casein are addictive.

Typically, some of the foods we've eaten all our life will be the most troublesome., and they will be the most difficult to eliminate from our diet. Some foods are actually addictive. The digestion of gluten and casein, for example, results in the production of gluteomorphins (also known as gliadorphins) and casomorphins.

These are actually opioid peptides, and they have a very addictive effect on the brain, similar to narcotics. This is why initially attempting to avoid gluten and casein can be very difficult, especially for some of us. Our brain actually craves gluten and casein after we have eaten them for so long. We have actually developed a dependency on them.

This is a big enough issue for some of us, that those who find avoiding these foods to be extremely difficult, may benefit from eliminating only one of them initially, and then eliminating the other after successfully eliminating the first one. Some of us find that changing our diet to control the disease is relatively easy, while others find it very difficult.

Changing our diet will change our gut biome.

Any time we change our diet, this will change the population distribution of the various bacteria in our intestines. Of course, our gut biome has already been altered by the development of MC. MC significantly compromises our digestion, which results in some foods being only partially digested.

As once previously mentioned, this occurs because the inflammation associated with MC interferes with the ability of our small intestine to produce the enzymes needed to digest various foods. Certain carbohydrates, and highly refined carbohydrates, tend to be especially difficult to digest. For many of us, the ability of our pancreas to produce digestive enzymes is also compromised because of the inflammation.

Opportunistic gut bacteria will take over.

Bacteria which thrive on the fermentation of partially digested food will tend to dominate, and they will largely replace the bacteria that previously populated our gut. After we begin to recover, and our digestion improves, these bacteria will be replaced by a more normal gut bacteria profile. But the main point is, our gut bacteria profile will always be specific to the foods in our diet, our ability to digest those foods efficiently, and the environment in which we live (which provides the microbe species available to us).

At this point, if the patient's doctor is a naturopath, the doctor will often diagnose the patient with small intestinal bacterial overgrowth (SIBO), and attempt to treat the SIBO, usually with antibiotics. But for the reasons stated in the previous paragraph, attempting to treat SIBO is futile, because in a week or two, our gut biome is going to revert right back to where it wants to be, based on our current diet, and our digestive efficiency.

As the saying goes, "Trying to fool mother nature is not nice". Yes, it's possible to treat SIBO, and doing so will temporarily alter the gut bacteria profile. But for most of us, this is a waste of time and money, because after a week or two, the gut bacteria profile will revert back to the biome that our diet and digestive ability currently enhances.

A recovery diet should be low-carb.

In chapter 2, we touched on the issue of compromised production of digestive enzymes, whenever the intestines are inflamed. This issue can even be noticed during periods of relatively short-term inflammation, such as a bout of the flu. When we have the flu, we immediately become short of the lactase enzyme, so we become temporarily lactose-intolerant. As we recover, and the inflammation fades away, we once again become able to digest lactose.

The problem of compromised enzyme production due to inflammation of the intestines is much more pronounced with the chronic inflammation associated with MC, and we eventually lose the ability to produce normal amounts of a number of different digestive enzymes because of the constant inflammation. Because this issue especially affects the digestion of certain carbohydrates, it's generally beneficial to choose low-carb foods in a recovery diet.

Protein heals, while certain certain carbs and other foods may interfere with healing.

The body uses protein to heal the damage caused by the inflammation, so greater than normal amounts of protein are needed in a recovery diet, to enhance healing. Carbohydrates, especially certain carbs and certain other foods, in larger amounts, tend to retard healing.

It was noted in chapter 2 how too much fiber can irritate the intestines, but other foods, and especially grains, can promote and perpetuate inflammation because of the lectins and other antinutrients they contain. A normal, healthy digestive system can usually tolerate the anti-nutrients in foods without significant problems. But when our gut is inflamed, we can recover our health much more quickly if we minimize these potential problems in our diet, by simply minimizing certain foods in our diet while we're recovering.

The anti-nutrients referred to here include (but are not limited to) lectins, chitins, benzoxazinoids, and amylase trypsin inhibitors (ATIs). The details of how those items compromise healing won't be covered here, because that's covered in my book, *Understanding Microscopic Colitis*, and other references. Suffice to say that they tend to promote leaky gut, so therefore, regularly eating foods that contain significant amounts of anti-nutrients, may initiate the creation of new food sensitivities, in some cases, and interfere with digestion, in others.

Why Sugar should be minimized during recovery.

Because of the reduction in the production of digestive enzymes mentioned above, due to the inflammation, only relatively small amounts of sugar can be properly digested. The rest of the partially digested sugar will pass into the colon, where it will probably be fermented by bacteria, producing gas, bloating, and sometimes, diarrhea. This doesn't result in the production of antibodies, but the symptoms can still be very uncomfortable.

A much bigger risk is leaky gut, due to excessive amounts of sugar.

A study done in Canada that used mice as subjects, showed that a diet high in sugar can not only cause increased intestinal permeability, but it can also compromise the functioning of the immune system, often leading to the development of colitis (Laffin, et al., 2019).[4] This potential problem appears to be generally supported by the experiences of many MC patients.

Certain starches are easier to digest than others.

There are basically two types of starch, amylose and amylopectin. All starchy foods contain a certain percentage of each type. Amylopectin starch is much easier to digest, but it is not soluble in water. Amylose starch is water-soluble. Foods with high amylose content are referred to as high starch foods, and foods with low amylose content are known as low starch foods.

Choose waxy foods, whenever they are an option.

Low starch foods contain high levels of amylopectin, and they're sometimes referred to as waxy foods. The bottom line here is that if we're looking for foods that will be easier to digest while we're recovering, we should choose waxy foods.

Avoid resistant starches.

Beware of foods that contain high levels of starches that are referred to as resistant starches, because resistant starches are not digestible by the human digestive system. Foods in this category are often promoted as diet foods, but they are definitely not friendly foods for MC patients, so they should be avoided when choosing foods for a recovery diet. Since our digestion is compromised by the disease, any foods that are difficult to digest, should definitely be avoided while trying to recover from MC.

Consider these examples of waxy foods.

Red potatoes are much easier to digest than russet potatoes, because russets are rated as high starch potatoes. Russets have a high amylose content. Red potatoes are considered to be waxy potatoes, because they have a high amylopectin content, placing them in the low starch category. Yukon gold potatoes are ranked as medium starch potatoes, so their digestibility lies about midway between the other two examples.

Waxy foods may be poor choices for diabetics.

Easy digestion means rapid digestion. With carbs, rapid digestion means a higher glycemic index, and this may be important to someone who has diabetes. Foods that contain higher amylose levels may be more difficult to digest, but they will prevent spikes in blood sugar, so this should be kept in mind whenever carbohydrates are being selected.

Similar rules apply to food such as rice.

Long grain rice cooks up fluffy, and doesn't tend to stick together, because it has a relatively high amylose content. But this makes it more difficult to digest. Short-grain rice is usually easier to digest, because it contains a higher percentage of amylopectin. Jasmine rice is an exception, because even though it's a long grain rice variety, it contains more amylopectin than most other long grain varieties. But the easiest rice to digest is waxy rice, or what's known as glutinous rice. This rice is usually grown in East or Southeast Asia. It contains the highest amylopectin percentage of all the rice varieties. But as with potatoes, waxy rice may not be a good choice for anyone who has diabetes.

There are even waxy corn varieties.

Unfortunately, very few foods are available that utilize waxy corn. Waxy corn is primarily used for making thickeners and stabilizers that are used as ingredients in certain foods. Waxy corn is available as bulk grain, however, so utilizing it might be an option for someone who makes their own corn tortillas, for example.

Poor digestion and malabsorption of nutrients are common problems during recovery.

Waxy foods should be considered by anyone who is having trouble digesting food, and absorbing nutrients from their food. After remission is attained, and the intestines have had time to heal for a while, waxy foods probably won't be needed for good digestion.

Here are a few specific details about the reactive peptides in gluten.

Gluten contains two primary protein fractions that have been shown to cause many people to react. These two fractions are prolamins, which are storage proteins, and glutelins. Although all grains contain their own unique forms of gluten, only the gluten in wheat and its close relatives, such as rye and barley, typically trigger reactions from celiacs and MC patients. Specifically, the prolamins in wheat are called gliadins, and the glutelins are called glutenins.

Anyone who is sensitive to these proteins, is also sensitive to the prolamins in rye and barley, which are known as secalin and hordein, respectively. And most of those individuals are also sensitive to the avenin prolamin in oats. Research has shown that when digested, altogether, these grains are known to be associated with several hundred different peptides that can trigger reactions in celiacs, and others (such as MC patients), who are sensitive to this group of grains (Tye-Din, et al., 2010).[5]

The only other grain for which a glutelin is commonly mentioned, is rice. That glutelin is known as orycenin. Only a very small percentage of people react to it, and it's not associated with celiac disease. Although some MC patients are sensitive to the zein in corn, zein is a prolamin protein, rather than a glutelin.

What about ancient grains?

The Internet contains more than a few blogs by misguided individuals who recommend using ancient grains to replace wheat in the diet. While there are a few examples of ancient grains that are safe substitutes for wheat, most of them contain gluten, and therefore, they are not safe, certainly not for MC patients, nor celiacs. They tend to contain smaller percentages of gluten, but for most MC patients, the gluten content is more than enough to trigger a reaction.

All of the grains produced today, including corn, sorghum, rice, wheat, and others, evolved from a common ancestor, which was a grass. But only the modern small grains that are more closely related to wheat, such as the ones mentioned on the previous page, share the reactive characteristics of wheat.

Safe, gluten-free ancient grains do exist.

A few of the ancient grains that evolved independently from wheat, are indeed free of gluten, as long as they're handled, processed, and stored carefully so that they don't become cross contaminated. Examples of these safe grains include millet, teff, amaranth, ragi, Job's tears, buckwheat, and quinoa (Kasarda, n.d.).[6] Ragi and Job's tears (which is also called adlay), are actually special varieties of millet. Although most of these have very tiny grain size, they're typically available as whole grains, and as flour.

Beware of other ancient grains promoted as gluten free.

Although other ancient grains that were not mentioned in the preceding paragraph are sometimes promoted as being gluten free, or safe for celiacs, please be aware that they are not. Often, they may have a significantly lower gluten content, but they are not gluten free, and continuing to eat them will result in reactions. In most such situations, the reactions will begin with the first exposure.

Malabsorption of certain vitamins and minerals is common when MC is active.

The secretory diarrhea caused by MC tends to deplete water-soluble vitamins and minerals. They are lost with the diarrhea, and tend to become depleted because nutrient absorption is compromised when the intestines are inflamed. Consequently, most MC patients become vitamin D and magnesium deficient after they have reacted for a while. This is important, because the immune system not only helps to prevent disease and infections, but it also controls healing. The immune system uses the active form of vitamin D when performing its duties, similar to the fuel on which an engine operates. And it must have an adequate amount of magnesium available, in order to enable the chemical conversion of the inactive form of vitamin D into the active form, so that the immune system can use it. Our food and supplements contain an inactive form of vitamin D.

Some patients are deficient before they develop the disease. A vitamin D or magnesium deficiency weakens the immune system, which is associated with an increased risk of developing MC, or some other disease. Because adequate amounts of vitamin D and magnesium are necessary in order that the immune system can perform properly, taking a vitamin D supplement will help healing. And if magnesium reserves are low, a magnesium supplement may be needed.

But significant amounts of magnesium can have laxative properties, and this varies by the type of magnesium supplement used. Some people are more sensitive to magnesium than others, especially while having an MC reaction. In such a situation, topical magnesium may be less likely to cause diarrhea, than an oral supplement. In this case, using a foot soak several times a week in which Epsom salts or magnesium chloride have been dissolved may help, or Epsom salts can be added to bathwater, and soaking for 15 or 20 minutes can be helpful. While this isn't as effective as an oral supplement, it's certainly better than nothing.

If I take a supplement, how much should I take?

Accurate vitamin D levels are easily measured by a simple blood test. Measuring magnesium reserves is a lot trickier, because most doctors mistakenly order a serum magnesium test, and less than 1% of the body's total magnesium is contained in blood serum, and that level is carefully regulated by the body within a narrow, normal range. Magnesium is a critical electrolyte that regulates cardiac activity and several other vital body functions. Consequently, serum levels of magnesium that are significantly

Issues to consider when selecting a recovery diet.

too high or too low can cause serious cardiac issues. Because of this, although serum magnesium test results may be valuable in an emergency department setting, this test is useless for routine determinations of magnesium reserves in the body. A much more accurate test for magnesium is the red blood cell (RBC) magnesium test. The RBC magnesium test measures the amount of magnesium in red blood cells, and that provides a much more accurate estimate of magnesium reserves in the cells of the body.

Therefore, if accurate vitamin D and magnesium test results are available, they may provide some insight into how much vitamin D or magnesium should be supplemented. In the absence of those test results, research shows that the average adult uses about 5000 international unit's (IU) of vitamin D daily, so this is an amount that can usually be safely taken until we have a chance to get accurate blood test results. It's generally safe to take this amount regardless of our situation. When the immune system is working overtime, as it is when it's dealing with an active MC reaction, a larger supplemental amount may be needed. But if we take significantly more than 5000 IU of vitamin D every day, we need to remember to have our vitamin D level tested after a few months, in case we don't need a higher dose of supplemental vitamin D. Ideally, a vitamin D level between 40 and 60 nanograms per milliliter (ng/mL) will help to heal the intestines.

As mentioned earlier, selecting a supplemental magnesium dose is more difficult. If we can tolerate it, the recommended daily allowance (RDA) of magnesium is a good, normally-safe dose. This would suggest about 400 mg for men, and about 300 mg for women. And this amount should be divided up throughout the day, with meals, in order to reduce the chances of it causing diarrhea. The body can only absorb and utilize a limited amount of magnesium at any given time, and any excess magnesium will remain in the intestines, where it can act as a laxative, especially in larger amounts of certain types of magnesium. Most MC patients find that they have the best results using magnesium glycinate, which is chelated magnesium. It tends to be easily absorbed, and appears to be one of the forms that is the least likely to cause diarrhea. But as mentioned previously, for those who can't tolerate an oral magnesium supplement, topical magnesium oil or lotion can be used.

Most nutrients are usually absorbed in the small intestine, but electrolyte are absorbed in the terminal ilium, and the colon. MC causes inflammation of the terminal ilium and the colon, and this often leads to other electrolyte issues such as a potassium deficiency. But it's best not to be concerned with this issue unless a doctor orders a test that shows you to be potassium deficient, and writes a prescription for a potassium supplement.

People who are magnesium deficient tend to have a difficult time absorbing magnesium, because published medical research shows that magnesium deficiency causes insulin resistance. Insulin resistance compromises the ability of the body to absorb and utilize nutrients, which of course includes magnesium. This makes retraining the body to be able to properly absorb magnesium quite difficult, because the insulin resistance must be overcome (by the restoration of magnesium reserves) before the normal absorption of any nutrients (including magnesium) will

Issues to consider when selecting a recovery diet.

resume. Since this is somewhat of a Catch-22 situation, regaining the ability to absorb magnesium can be a slow process, that has to be initiated slowly. This appears to be the primary reason why MC patients especially, have varying degrees of the ability to absorb magnesium, and why it can cause significant problems for some individuals.

Summary
In order to reach remission from the symptoms of the disease, we have to avoid all (not just most) of the foods that are causing our immune system to produce antibodies. We must also minimize fiber and sugar in the diet, because although they don't cause the production of antibodies, they tend to irritate our intestines, which can slow down recovery. Gluten and casein are especially difficult for many people to avoid, because when digested, they produce opioids, that can be as addictive as narcotics.

Our gut biome changes as our digestive capabilities change. Additionally, certain medications, and any diet changes, will change the composition of our gut biome. Some types of foods are much easier to digest than others, especially when our MC is active, and our digestion is compromised.

Chapter 4

Choosing safe foods for a recovery diet

We've discussed the foods that must be avoided, and the reasons why they must be avoided in a recovery diet. Now let's consider foods that are safe to include in a recovery diet. Interestingly, less common foods, or foods that we normally don't eat, tend to be safer choices than foods we've been eating all our lives.

The food choices specified here are for an elimination diet.

Unless otherwise specified, the food choices outlined here will be choices that should be made for an elimination diet. In other words, these selections should be made whenever EnteroLab. test results are not available. If the appropriate EnteroLab tests are ordered, any foods shown to be safe by those results, can also be included in the safe food options.

Bear in mind that a recovery diet must contain foods that are essential for good health. That means that a recovery diet must include protein and fat. That said, because fat malabsorption is a common problem whenever MC is active (causing a reaction, fat must usually be limited in a recovery diet. A larger than normal amount of protein is necessary, because protein is required for healing. And at least a minimal amount of fat must be included in order to prevent what's known as rabbit starvation, or protein poisoning. A diet without sufficient fat can cause diarrhea and other digestive symptoms within about a week.

Carbohydrates are optional in a recovery diet.

Carbs are not required for good health, despite the implications of many online health blogs. If carbs are selected, vegetables are preferred sources, rather than grains and fruits, and they should be peeled and overcooked. Safe vegetable choices for most of us include carrots, squash, rutabaga, cauliflower, sweet potatoes, yams, and similar vegetables. Green beans are normally safe when properly cooked, despite the fact that they are legumes.

Whole (mature) beans, on the other hand, should be avoided, especially in a recovery diet. Although foods such as broccoli, cabbage, and some of the other crucibles are usually safe, normally they are best avoided during recovery, because their digestion produces a significant amount of gas, and most of us have a problem eliminating gas, while we are recovering.

Dark green leafy vegetables, such as spinach, should be avoided, at least in larger servings, due to their relatively large oxalate content. A small amount is usually not a problem, but larger amounts may cause digestive problems, gout, and kidney stones for some individuals. Iceberg lettuce should be totally avoided in an elimination diet, and raw salads, in general, should be eliminated until well after remission is achieved.

Resist the temptation to eat gluten-free bread.

Most MC patients attempt to find a substitute for bread, and they usually choose one of the commercially produced gluten-free bread products. But the problem with virtually all of those bread products is the fact that they all contain far too many ingredients to be a safe option. Almost invariably, there will be one or more ingredients in them that most of us cannot tolerate, and while eating a slice or two of that bread may not cause an immediate reaction, it may be inflammatory enough to prevent us from reaching remission. So why take a chance on never reaching remission? After we're in remission, and we've acquired some healing, many of us are able to tolerate -most brands of these breads. But it's definitely best to wait until we've been in stable remission for a while, before trying to add a gluten-free bread to our diet.

Vegan, or vegetarian diet issues.

MC patients following a vegan, or vegetarian lifestyle, may not be able to find a safe protein source within the restrictions of those lifestyles, unless they're fortunate enough to not be sensitive to soy. Unfortunately, that is seldom the case, because most MC patients are sensitive to soy, and a sensitivity to soy typically includes sensitivity to most legumes.

The preferred protein choice is meat.

Meat is the best protein choice, because it contains all the essential amino acids required for good health. Meat from wild animals or wild -type animals that have been raised on farms or ranches, are typically safe for everyone. This includes turkey, duck, goose, pheasant, quail, emu, venison, lamb, goat, antelope, and rabbit, for example. Notice that bison are not included in this list, because these days, most bison contain DNA from domestic cattle, due to crossbreeding, over the decades.

Shellfish are usually safe options.

Shellfish, including muscles, clams, oysters, shrimp, prawns, and others, are also usually safe for everyone, except for those who had a shellfish allergy before they developed MC. Some fish species may be safe, but many of us react to certain fish, consequently, fish are best avoided as choices for a recovery diet. If desired, after remission is achieved, they can be tested to see if they're a safe option.

Is it safe to drink coffee?

Coffee is a secretagog, meaning that it causes increased secretions, and because of that, most gastroenterologists advise MC patients not to drink coffee. Regardless, most MC patients can continue to drink coffee without any problems, provided that they didn't have to rush to the bathroom as soon as they drank a cup of coffee, before they developed MC. Because this is not true for everyone, it's safer to avoid coffee until after remission is achieved. After stable remission is reached, coffee can be tested, and added back into the diet, if it doesn't seem to be a problem (and it isn't, for most of us).

Beware of so-called nondairy creamers.

Do not add milk to your coffee., not even a nondairy creamer, because many nondairy creamers contain derivatives of casein.

Choosing safe foods for a recovery diet

The manufacturers of those products mistakenly assume that most dairy intolerance is is due to lactose intolerance. While we are indeed lactose intolerant any time our intestines are inflamed, lactose does not cause the production of antibodies by our immune system.

The primary problem with products made from milk, is the casein content. All dairy products contain casein, and casein causes our immune system to produce antibodies against it, if we're sensitive to casein. All of us are lactose intolerant(whenever our intestines are inflamed), and most of us have a casein sensitivity. If you prefer to add anything to your coffee, add ordinary cane sugar, or a nut milk (if you're not sensitive to these nuts) such as almond milk, cashew milk, or coconut milk. When using coconut milk, choosing refined coconut milk is usually preferred, since refining removes virtually all of the coconut taste, however, beware of inflammatory additives. Again, coffee is best avoided during recovery. It's much safer to add coffee to your diet after you're in remission.

Be very careful about selecting foods for a recovery diet.

Above all, remember that if any food is selected for a recovery diet, and that food causes our immune system to produce antibodies, we may never be able to achieve remission. A recovery diet must be simple, bland, and consist of only a few basic, safe foods, in order to minimize the risk of unintentionally including a food that causes us to react. In other words, the fewer foods a recovery diet includes, the lower the risk of failure; consequently, the higher the odds that the diet will successfully bring remission.

Our previous diet is history.

Attempting to design a recovery diet by simply avoiding certain foods, or by selecting alternative foods that mimic our previous diet, is often not successful. Rather, a recovery diet should be designed from scratch, by selecting only safe foods. The fewer the number of foods in that diet, the sooner we are normally able to reach remission, and the lower the risk of accidentally including a food that may prevent us from ever reaching remission.

Our food is our medicine.

Remember that a recovery diet is the medicine that we have chosen to treat our disease. Accordingly, we shouldn't expect it to be an epicurean treat. That's not our goal. Our goal is to get the symptoms of our disease under control by stopping the inflammation, so that our intestines can heal, and allow us to achieve long-term remission.

After we're safely in remission, and our intestines have healed for a while, we can test the safety of new foods, and various seasonings, one at a time, of course, before we add them into our diet. After we're in remission, we will once again begin to regain the ability to properly digest foods, and as our digestive system heals, we'll be able to slowly add enhancements that will make our meals much more enjoyable.

Breakfasts can be challenging.

But during recovery, when normal breakfast foods are not known to be safe, breakfast can look like any other meal. In other words, a good choice may be leftovers from dinner or lunch the day before. Of course, if EnteroLab test results are available, and they show chicken eggs and pork to be safe, then eggs and bacon would be safe breakfast selections. But without those test results, it's safer by far to avoid those foods until remission is attained, and then they can be tested for safety.

If you should find yourself without leftovers, or any other options, consider something like hash brown potatoes and your choice of meat. Very few of us are sensitive to potatoes. Obviously, don't try this, if you know that you're sensitive to potatoes.

Most breakfast cereals contain barley malt. Consequently, they contain gluten. Many also contain soy. And most breakfast cereals contain far too many ingredients, which make them a risky choice. Fortunately, safe cereals do exist, but they should be avoided during recovery. Once remission is gained, breakfast cereals such as Corn Chex and Rice Chex can be tested for safety. But during recovery, cereals such as these contain far too many ingredients to be automatically considered safe for most MC patients (especially during recovery).

Eating out should be avoided.

Especially during recovery, eating away from home, should be avoided. Research studies show that over half the meals served at restaurants that are claimed to be gluten-free, are not.. Contamination rates tend to be lower in the mornings, and significantly higher late in the day, suggesting that countertops are not cleaned regularly during the day, or possibly restaurant workers may become more careless as the day wears on. And if foods served in restaurants tend to be cross contaminated with gluten, it's also a pretty safe bet that they may be cross contaminated with casein and soy, as well.

Regardless of the cause, breakfasts served at restaurants tend to be significantly safer than dinners served in the evening. It should be obvious that a 50% cross-contamination rate is totally unacceptable for anyone who ever hopes to reach remission.

High end restaurants are much safer choices.

If you must eat out, try to choose a high-end restaurant, if possible. Their chefs understand how to prepare meals that are allergen free, as long as you make your needs clear to the waiter or waitress.

Eating at friends and relatives' homes is also risky.

As you will soon discover, if you haven't already, learning how to avoid even traces of risky ingredients when preparing our meals, is not a simple matter. It takes time to learn all the details well enough to avoid making mistakes. Therefore, unless someone has experience in preparing meals for a family member who has celiac disease, or some other food sensitivity issue, it's best to assume that despite their insistence to the contrary, they probably are not capable of preparing food without a significant risk of cross-contamination. In such a situation, volunteering to do the cooking, may be a practical solution. And in doing so, you will have the opportunity to show them how to go about cooking safe meals, so that in the future, if the need arises, they will know how to prepare allergen free meals.

Traveling requires careful planning.

When traveling by automobile, many individuals with food sensitivities take an ice chest, or a small portable refrigerator that will plug into a 12 volt receptacle. This allows them to take their meals with them, so that at their destination, they can simply warm-up their foods with a microwave oven. Meals and snacks can be prepared prior to the trip, and stored in plastic bags.

Traveling by air is more difficult.

If an airline is contacted at least two weeks before your trip, they can serve at least gluten-free meals, although they may not be familiar with other food allergies. However, please be aware that most airlines' idea of a gluten-free meal is fruit or a similar cold snack. Some MC patients take their meals with them. However, they must be properly packed, especially liquids, in order to get through security inspections. Consulting ahead of time, with a friend who has experience with this, such as someone who has food sensitivities and travels a lot, can make the job much easier.

Cooking in large batches saves time

Cooking foods in relatively large batches, and dividing it into meal size portions can make life much easier in the long run, and prevent situations where we have nothing safe available to eat. The servings can then be stored in individual plastic containers (or plastic bags) in a deep-freeze, and a package can be taken out and warmed up, or microwaved, whenever it's needed.

Bone broth helps healing

Homemade bone broth helps intestinal healing. It's a great source of nutrients, such as vitamins, minerals, and collagen. It can be sipped as a drink during the day, poured over food as a sauce, to add flavor, or even used as the liquid when cooking vegetables or other foods, such as rice. And, of course, it makes a great base for stews or soups. All we need to do is add vegetables and our choice of meat, season to taste (using safe seasoning), and simmer. Obviously we'll need to cook it longer, if the meat and vegetables are raw.

Any leftover bones from meats that are safe for us will make good bone broth. Chicken, duck, or turkey carcasses can be used. Beef, lamb, pork, or venison bones, for example, especially when they include joints, make good bone broth. Even chicken feet can be used. Just fill a large pot about three-quarter full of water, add the bones, and a little salt, and boil for a few hours. Or, it can be simmered in a crockpot for about 12 to 24 hours. Some people cook bone broth for four to six hours, while others cook it much longer. Some add apple cider vinegar. We can use whatever technique appeals to us.

When we've finished cooking, we can remove the bones, and divide the broth into smaller containers, and store it in the deep--freeze until needed. If it seems to gel as it cools, that simply means that it contains a significant amount of collagen.

Are you searching for a mid-morning or mid-afternoon snack?

Here's a tasty idea that works for most people. Peel bananas and store them in plastic bags in the deep-freeze. When we crave a snack, we can take one out and let it partially thaw for about a minute or so. Or we can eat it immediately, if we prefer. Don't overdo the thawing time, or the banana will become too mushy.

When it's ready to eat, we can put a little cashew butter, almond butter, or some other nut butter we've found to be safe, on the end of the banana, and take a bite. We can use whatever amount appeals to us, and add a little nut butter each time, before we take a bite. Most people find this to be much tastier than a Popsicle, and obviously it makes a much healthier snack.

Bananas are a high histamine food.

But if we happen to have histamine problems, bananas, may not be a safe option. The riper bananas get, the higher the histamine level becomes. For those who have histamine problems, a frozen banana may be tolerable for an occasional snack if it's frozen before it becomes completely ripe (or even when it's a little on the green side). Also, we should be aware that most nuts, and therefore most nut butters , may be high histamine foods, so we may need to limit our intake of them (assuming that we can tolerate them, in the first place).

61

For those in remission, raw apples should be safe.

A fresh, peeled, sliced apple can be eaten this way, instead of a frozen banana. Apples are not a high histamine food. The nut butter adds protein and flavor. And, of course, peanut butter could be used with either of these fruits, but peanut butter must be avoided by anyone who is sensitive to soy. However, raw apples should be avoided by those who are still not in remission. Peeled, overcooked apples, are an option for those not yet in remission, but the serving size should be limited in order to avoid exceeding the amount of fiber in the diet that we can tolerate.

We should always test any "new" foods before adding them into our diet.

After remission is attained, before any foods are added to our diet, they should be tested by trial and error, one at a time, by starting with a small helping, and then eating a progressively larger helping each day, for up to three days. Testing of a food should be stopped if it causes a reaction at any time. But if no reaction is detected after three days of eating a food, then that food can usually be safely added into our diet.

Summary

We should avoid commercially processed products while recovering — they typically contain too many ingredients, so that even if the individual ingredients appear to be safe, the combination of ingredients often causes MC patients to react. And we should avoid eating out while on a recovery diet, because research shows that most restaurant food claimed to be gluten-free, is not. Consequently, it's very likely that restaurant food also contains other food ingredients that we must avoid. And despite their best intentions, meals prepared by friends and relatives are typically unsafe for MC patients, unless they been specially trained to understand the details of preparing safe foods.

Chapter 5

Vitamins, Minerals, and Methylation Issues

The immune system is in charge of healing any and all damage to any organ in the body. Most damaged cells are replaced by new cells, but when they can't be replaced by new cells, they're replaced by scar tissue. The only organs in the body in which the cells cannot normally be replaced by new cells are the heart and the brain.

Most cells are replaced on some predetermined schedule, or if they should become damaged. Because of all the wear and tear caused by the digestion of food, cells in the lining of the digestive tract are replaced with new cells more frequently than the cells in most other organs. Normally, they're replaced on a weekly basis in the intestines, and even more frequently in the lining of the stomach.

Therefore, it's the immune system's responsibility to heal the damage that the inflammation caused by food sensitivies causes to the lining (epithelium) of the intestines. But because additional damage is incurred due to antibodies produced by food sensitivities in every meal, healing can never be completed (as long as we continue to eat those foods). This perpetuates the inflammation, and causes the disease to becomes chronic.

Every cell in the body has a vitamin D receptor.

Obviously, vitamin D must be very important. Optimal healing requires optimal immune system functionality, and this requires relatively high levels of the active form of vitamin D, 1,25(OH)2D (aka 1,25-dihydroxyvitamin D) in the cells to be healed. Also, adequate magnesium is required in order to activate the methylation process (defined on the next page) that allows the inactive form of vitamin D to be converted into the active form.

While vitamin D, and frequently magnesium, tend to be the only supplements that are advised to be taken during recovery, after remission is achieved, additional vitamins and mineral supplements should be considered, if one's long-term maintenance diet is deficient of any vitamins or minerals. For most of us, our long-term diet will probably provide adequate nutrition. But some diets are so restricted that vitamin and mineral supplements may be needed.

Unfortunately, many of us are unable to utilize common vitamin supplements.

If vitamin supplements are needed, the process of selecting the supplements may be complicated by the fact that more than half of us are unable to properly utilize vitamins in their normal forms because of certain genetic mutations. The vitamins in food and most over-the-counter supplements are in their inactive forms. These are stable forms, so that they don't quickly lose their nutritional value. Supplements have a significantly lower cost, and they're able to provide maximum shelf life when they're in their inactive forms. But our body requires vitamins in the active forms in order for our immune system and our organs to be able to utilize them. The biochemical process by which the body converts vitamins from the inactive forms into the active forms, involves a chemical conversion known as a methylation process.

Methylation is a simple biochemical process.

It involves the transfer of one carbon and three hydrogen atoms (CH3) between two chemical compounds. In the body, CH3 is supplied by SAMe (S-adenosylmethionine). But the production of SAMe depends upon the availability of 5-methyltetrahydro-folate (5-MTHF), which is the active form of folate, known as methylfolate, and about 60% of us have one or more genetic mutations that compromise our ability to carry out the methyla-tion process that allows folate to be converted into methylfolate. Scaglione, and Panzavolta. (2014) point out that, "Folate defi-ciency has been linked with an increased risk of neural tube defects, cardiovascular disease, cancer and cognitive dysfunc-tion."[7]

MTHFR gene mutations cause methylation issues.

The methylation process is regulated by methylenetetrahydrofo-late reductase (MTHFR) enzyme, and the production of this enzyme is encoded by the MTHFR gene. When mutations of this gene occur, the methylation process can be compromised in a variety of different ways, depending upon the nature of the mutations. As noted above, approximately 60% of us have one or more genetic mutations that interfere with our ability to complete this conversion normally, and this can frustrate our body's ability to utilize ordinary vitamins. Depending upon the extent of our MTHFR gene mutations, we may derive little to no benefit from ordinary, over the counter vitamin supplements. It's necessary for most of us who have MTHFR gene mutations to select vitamins that are available in the active (methylated) forms.

Fortified foods may provide limited vitamin benefits.

Although many foods are fortified with certain vitamins, including folic acid, if we have MTHFR gene mutations, we may not be able to utilize the vitamins that we believe to be in those foods. Likewise, we may not be able to utilize the natural folate content of leafy green vegetables, legumes, citrus fruits, and other foods. If we have one or more MTHFR gene mutations, and we ask our doctor to order tests to determine our vitamin levels, those test results will typically show high, or even above normal range levels for some of those vitamins, although our body is deficient in the active forms of those vitamins, and desperately in need of them.

Thorne Research, (n.d.), recommends the following 7 essential nutrients to assist in proper methylation for those who have methylation issues resulting from MTHFR gene mutations.[8]

Vitamins, Minerals, and Methylation Issues

1. 5-MTHF (active folate)
2. Methylcobalamin (active vitamin B12)
3. Pyridoxal 5'-Phosphate (active vitamin B6)
4. Riboflavin 5'-Phosphate (active vitamin B2)
5. Magnesium
6. Betaine (also known as trimethylglycine)
7. Vitamin D

Thorne Research produces a dietary supplement called Methyl-Guard that contains 5 MTHF (folate), methylcobalamin (B12), Pyridoxal 5'-Phosphate (B6), and betaine. In addition, they produce another product called Methyl-Guard Plus that contains higher doses of all those ingredients, plus riboflavin (B2).

The 2 products mentioned above are generics for a prescription vitamin supplement.

The prescription-only pharmaceutical product known as Metanx is often prescribed by doctors for diabetes patients to treat nerve damage caused by diabetes mellitus. Metanx contains 5 MTHF (folate, methylcobalamin (B12), and Pyridoxal 5'-Phosphate (B6). Of course the prescription medication Metanx is significantly more expensive than the over-the-counter supplements sold by Thorne Research. More than a few people who may or may not have methylation issues, take Metanx, or one of the generic supplements, in order to enhance their cognitive abilities.

MTHFR gene mutations may cause issues with toxins and heavy metals.

Depending upon the extent of MTHFR gene mutations, the body's ability to break down and eliminate toxins and heavy metals tends to be compromised, which of course, can allow them to build up in the body. And the inability to properly convert folate or folic acid into methylfolate tends to allow a buildup of homocysteine, which is known to increase the risk of cardiovascular issues and dementia.

The take-home message here is, "If you have health issues that appear to be related to vitamin deficiencies, or you've had your vitamin levels tested, and you found that some of them are at the high-end of the normal range, or even above the normal range, you may have MTHFR gene mutations that are causing methylation issues."

Vitamin D

The Institute of Medicine's recommendations for vitamin D are 600–800 IUs daily, and they advise against taking more than 4,000 IUs per day. But that upper limit is simply there because there hasn't been enough published medical research to prove exactly what happens at higher dosage levels. At least there hasn't been enough published medical research based on random controlled trials (RCTs) to satisfy the strict criteria of the medical community.

But that doesn't mean that higher doses have been shown to be harmful. Actually, there have been more than a few studies proving that higher doses of vitamin D can be very beneficial, both for preventing the development of many diseases, especially autoimmune diseases, and for helping to treat those diseases. That implies that vitamin D enhances the effectiveness of the immune system, since the immune system is responsible not only for disease prevention, but also for healing.

How much vitamin D would be an overdose?

If we review the data, it's apparent that the only official recorded instances of honest-to-goodness cases of vitamin D overdose were associated with a daily dose of 40,000 IU or more that was ingested for at least several months. No evidence exists to show that taking that amount for a few days, or even for a few weeks is harmful. Nor is there any evidence that taking smaller amounts, such as 10,000 or 20,000 IUs for any length of time has been shown to be harmful.

IBDs deplete vitamin D.

While no dedicated studies have been done on the association of vitamin D levels and MC, studies have shown that Crohn's disease patients have lower levels of inflammation, and generally enjoy a better quality of life, when they have a higher vitamin D serum level. One study was done using Crohn's disease patients who were in remission. Some of the patients took 1,000 IU of vitamin D daily, and others took 10,000 IU of vitamin D daily (Narula, Cooray, Anglin, Muqtadir, Narula, & Marshall, 2017).[9] After a year-long study, those taking 10,000 IU of vitamin D daily had fewer relapses, and improved anxiety and depression scores.

71

Presumably, those taking the higher dose had improved outcomes because they had less inflammation, and less intestinal permeability (leaky gut). This implies that MC patients should generally enjoy the same level of improvement with higher vitamin D levels, since inflammation and increased intestinal permeability are responsible for causing most of the symptoms associated with the disease.

A number of these research articles suggest that hydroxy vitamin D [25(0H)D] serum levels in the range of 40–70 ng/ml (100–175 nmol/L) appear to be optimal for enhanced immune system functionality (Raftery and O'Sullivan, 2015).[10] And therefore, they should provide better results for patients who have an autoimmune disease.

Common knowledge says that vitamin D is activated in 2 stages. The liver converts vitamin D into 25-hydroxyvitamin D [25(OH)D], which is circulated in the blood. And the kidneys convert the 25(OH)D into the active form, 1,25(OH)2D (1,25-dihydroxyvitamin D). But the transformation into the active form can also take place locally (inside the cells).

Dr. Michael F Holick points out that virtually every cell in the body is capable of activating vitamin D locally (Taub, Manson, & Holick, 2021, December 01).[11] This suggests that all cells may be capable of completing other, possibly all, methylation processes locally, as well.

Magnesium

Magnesium and **insulin** are codependent. This means that whenever nutrients have been absorbed from the digestive system into the bloodstream, both insulin and magnesium are needed to transport the nutrients from the blood to the cells in the body wherever they're needed.

Taking a vitamin D supplement will increase the absorption of calcium, and since calcium is a critical electrolyte, the presence of the additional calcium in the blood requires that magnesium must either be used to help insulin to transport the calcium to the bones and other cells in the body where it's needed, or magnesium is required to purge the excess calcium from the bloodstream. Therefore, calcium depletes magnesium.

This implies that whenever a vitamin D supplement is taken, a magnesium supplement should also be taken. Published research shows that magnesium is used in over 300 chemical conversions that take place in the body every day, making adequate magnesium an essential requirement for good long-term health.

Selecting an oral magnesium supplement should be done carefully.

Pure magnesium, especially in the form of a fine powder, is so combustible that it's explosive. Because of that issue, oral magnesium supplements always contain magnesium compounded with another element, so that it will be in a stable form. But unfortunately, some forms are difficult to absorb. We can only absorb about 3 or 4% of the magnesium in magnesium oxide tablets, for example. The rest remains in the intestines, where it acts as a laxative, making magnesium oxide a very poor choice as a supplement, but a good choice for someone looking for a laxative.

At the other extreme, some chelated forms of magnesium are well absorbed, with a minimal risk of acting as a laxative. Magnesium glycinate, for example, is an excellent choice for most. MC patients. Some MC patients are able to absorb magnesium much better than others, so the optimal dose for individuals may vary, but a dose based on the RDA is almost always safe, and usually effective. The current RDA for women is 320 mg, and the RDA for men is 400 mg. Obviously an optimal dose will depend on the amount of magnesium in an individual's selected long-term diet, so if our diet contains relatively high amounts of magnesium, then any chosen magnesium supplement can be reduced accordingly.

Difficulty sleeping, or staying asleep, and especially waking up in the middle of the night with leg or foot cramps, indicates a chronic magnesium deficiency, and taking a magnesium supplement before bedtime will help us to to get more beneficial sleep, by relaxing our muscles.

The "B" vitamins

Vitamins B-12 and B-9

Vitamins, Minerals, and Methylation Issues

The B vitamins are essential for maintaining good immune system and nervous system health. The body can store vitamin B-12 reserves for up to about 5 years, normally, but the other B vitamins have no stored reserves. Active MC, or any active disease that causes high rates of diarrhea, tends to deplete water-soluble vitamins such as the B vitamins. Many MC patients will normally still have adequate B-12 reserves available, unless they react longer than 5 years before getting the disease under control.

That said, while vitamin B-12 is readily available in animal-based foods, plant-based diets contain very little vitamin B-12. Therefore, anyone following a vegan or vegetarian lifestyle will eventually become B-12 deficient, unless they take a vitamin B-12 supplement. Since folate is needed in order for the body to utilize B-12, whenever a B-12 vitamin supplement is taken, a B-9 (folate) vitamin supplement should also be taken.

MC patients often seek treatment for depression.

Note that recently published research shows that a vitamin B-12 deficiency is associated with an increased risk of depression (Trinity College Dublin, 2021, December 14).[12] It's well known that depression is a common symptom among many MC patients. While it's true that MC is indeed, a depressing disease, because of its embarrassing, and sometimes debilitating, symptoms, perhaps B-12 deficiency is more common among MC patients than conventional wisdom dictates.

MC patients who have refractive MC, or methylation issues, should take vitamin B supplements in the active forms, which would be methylcobalamin rather than the inactive form, cyanocobalamin, in the case of B-12, and 5-methyltetrahydrofolate (5-MTHF), rather than folic acid, in the case of B-9.

If we should decide to ask our doctor to order a test to measure our B-12 level, and we're currently taking a B-12 supplement, we need to stop taking it at least 10 days before having the blood draw for the test, or our result is likely to be unrealistically high. The level will be distorted until the various forms of B-12 in the body reach equilibrium (which may take up to about 10 days).

Vitamin B-6

Vitamin B-6 is known as pyridoxine when in the inactive form, and pyridoxal 5'-phosphate (P5P) when in the active form. Vitamin B–6 is required for at least 100 chemical processes that take place in the body on a daily basis.

One of the more important functions of vitamin B-6 is to promote the production of diamine oxidase (DAO) enzyme. IBD's tend to deplete DAO, and DAO is used by the body to purge excess (unused) histamine. If DAO drops to significantly below normal levels, the level of unused histamine tends to build up until eventually, histamine reactions are triggered. These reactions typically include the development of a rash and itching, which can eventually become a severe problem. MC patients who have methylation issues may need to take the active form of B-6, pyridoxal 5' phosphate.

Normally, the other B vitamins do not tend to become deficient for MC patients, according to published medical research data. However, although the mainstream medical community does not recognize vitamin B-2 (riboflavin) to be associated with MC, or any other IBD, it might possibly play a role in the fatigue that is so common with active MC.

Vitamin B-2

Vitamin B-2 facilitates the ability of the body to use the energy in fats, proteins, and carbs in the diet. Note that a vitamin B-2 deficiency is most commonly caused by anorexia and alcoholism. The cause of vitamin deficiencies due to anorexia is quite obvious, and unrelated to MC. Interestingly though, the cause of vitamin B-2 deficiency due to alcoholism is increased intestinal permeability (leaky gut). Because leaky gut is a common symptom of MC, that suggests that a B-2 deficiency might be common among MC patients, despite the fact that the medical community overlooks this possibility.

The take-home message here is that a vitamin B-2 supplement may be beneficial for some MC patients. Note that as mentioned in the discussion about methylation, Thorne Research manufactures a product that contains the active forms of vitamins B-12, B–9, B-6, and B-2, making this a very convenient way for MC patients, especially those who have methylation issues, to supplement all the B vitamins that may be needed.

Vitamin E

Vitamin E supplements are derived from many different sources, and many foods are enriched with various types of vitamin E, some of which are used as preservatives. Tracking down the source materials used to make the various forms of vitamin E often tends to be difficult. For example, vitamin E is often listed on labels as d-alpha tocopherol, dl-tocopherol, alpha tocopherol acetate, tocopherol acetate, mixed tocotrienols and vitamin E succinate. Some of these are natural forms, and some are artificial. These classifications certainly aren't obvious.

Vitamin E from natural sources occurs in 8 different chemical forms (isomers):

- Alpha tocopherol
- beta tocopherol
- delta tocopherol
- gamma tocopherol
- alpha tocotrienol
- beta tocotrienol
- delta tocotrienol
- gamma tocotrienol

It's generally acknowledged that only alpha tocopherol fulfills human nutritional requirements (Office of Dietary Supplements, n.d.).[13] Natural vitamin E supplements tend to contain only alpha tocopherol and it's listed on labels as d alpha-tocopherol. Although this is clearly the most beneficial form for vitamin E supplements, unfortunately, most of the natural vitamin E supplements available on the market, are derived from soy oil.

Many vitamin E supplements are synthetic.

Because it's cheaper to make synthetic vitamin E supplements, most of the vitamin E supplements on the market contain all 8 isomers (although the human body doesn't even utilize four of them), and this is designated on the label as dl-alpha-tocopherol. Research shows that the vast majority of synthetic vitamin E supplements are only about half as effective as natural forms of vitamin E.

But vitamin supplements do not include an important isomer.

Note that research shows that gamma tocopherol is actually the most common isomer found in food (roughly 70%), making it the elephant in the room, although most vitamin E supplements, whether they are natural or synthetic, do not include it (Jiang, Christen, Shigenaga, and Ames, 2001).[14] The fact that this isomer is predominant in food, but totally ignored in vitamin E supplements, raises the possibility that vitamin supplements may do more harm than good in some cases.

The problem is, when only alpha tocopherol is supplemented, this tends to deplete gamma tocopherol levels in the body. And this can lead to problems, because the body needs gamma tocopherol to reduce inflammation levels and enhance protection against certain diseases, including certain cancers. Gamma tocopherol has also been shown to activate genes that are protective against Alzheimer's disease.

Are vitamin E supplements actually useful?

The exclusion of gamma tocopherol raises the possibility that no type of vitamin E supplement, whether natural or synthetic, is likely to be beneficial for improving protection levels against certain diseases. This obviously leaves foods (not enriched foods), as the best source of beneficial vitamin E. Good food sources of vitamin E include (but are certainly not limited to) almonds, avocados, broccoli, fish, olive oil, safflower oil, sunflower seeds and oil, spinach and other dark green leafy vegetables, squash, shellfish, and a few other foods. Most of these foods are well tolerated by most MC patients. Of course peanuts, soy and soy oil, and tomatoes contain high levels of vitamin E also, but many MC patients cannot tolerate them.

Most MC patients are less concerned about getting enough vitamin E, than they are about accidentally ingesting a form that was derived from soy. And to complicate matters, most manufacturers assume that vitamin D derived from soy oil should be labeled as soy free, because the proteins were all removed when the oil was refined. But unfortunately, refining is not a perfect process, and a very small fraction of one percent of soy proteins remain in the oil. While this doesn't necessarily apply to all of us, many of us tend to react to those very low levels of contamination.

Avoid d-tocopherol.

The take-home message here is, whenever natural forms of vitamin E are used (d-tocopherol), and the actual source of the ingredient is not specified as something other than soy, it's usually best to assume that the vitamin E was made from soy, because it's very unlikely that soy is indeed the source. As mentioned earlier, if the vitamin E is listed on the label as dl alpha-tocopherol, or as synthetic vitamin E, then it does not contain soy.

Beware of extracts, also.

Be careful with products that contain extracts, also because more often than not, soy oil is used as the extraction medium. For example many processed turkeys contain rosemary extract. While rosemary itself should not cause any problems, the extraction process is usually done with soy oil, and so rosemary extract may contain traces of soy protein, which can cause problems for many of us who are sensitive to soy.

Magnesium helps for getting better sleep.

If you have trouble sleeping, or staying asleep, and especially if you wake up in the middle of the night with leg or foot cramps, you may have a chronic magnesium deficiency, and taking a magnesium supplement before bedtime will help your muscles to relax, and allow you to get more beneficial sleep.

Always try to minimize stress.

Since stress is a big contributor to inflammation, and it raises our anxiety level and prevents our brain from relaxing, doing something relaxing, such as reading, or listening to relaxation recordings, or pursuing a favorite hobby for a while before going to bed is a much better way to prepare ourselves for restful sleep, than watching the news on TV, for example.

Summary

Most MC patients are vitamin D and magnesium deficient. Most of us also have MTHFR gene mutations that cause methylation issues, so that our bodies have varying degrees of difficulty converting inactive vitamin forms into the active forms, so that our immune system and other cellular chemical processes that take place in the body, can use them.

Chapter 6

Meal Suggestions

As a general rule, we need to eat some protein with every meal or snack to encourage healing, and to reduce the tendency to be hungry again within a couple of hours. During recovery, it's better to eat smaller meals more frequently, than to eat two or three big meals each day. This helps to improve digestion, because it minimizes the possibility of running out of digestive enzymes before we're able to finish digesting a meal. First, since this is the most difficult diet selection situation, we'll consider meals for those who are sensitive to all of the foods tested by EnteroLab, including gluten, casein (cow's milk), soy, chicken eggs, beef, pork, chicken, tuna, corn, rice, oats, walnut, cashew, almond, and white potato.

Choosing foods when we seem to react to all foods.

Except for nontypical situations, the EnteroLab test panels A1 + C1 include tests for all foods that typically cause reactions for MC patients. Conversely, foods not included in these test panels normally do not trigger reactions for MC patients, so most of us can assume that they are safe selections for a recovery diet.

"What can I eat?"

Patients in this situation usually ask, "But what can I eat?", as if there are no options left for them. The EnteroLab test panels only test for sensitivity to 11 foods. But as pointed out above, these are the only foods that are commonly associated with reactions due to microscopic colitis. Are there only 11 foods in the world? Certainly not, so obviously, there are many remaining possibilities from which to select a safe diet. In other words we need to select foods that previously were not usually a part of our diet.

While it's true that in certain cases, some MC patients do react to other foods, this is very atypical, and those reactions may be associated with other health issues, rather than due to MC. Obviously, if you know that you react to certain foods, regardless of the cause, continue to avoid those foods.

Safe protein selections

The safest protein options will be meats that we do not regularly eat, such as turkey, quail, duck, goose, emu, lamb, cabrito (goat), venison, antelope, rabbit, and similar choices. Also, unless we were previously allergic to them, shellfish are usually safe for most of us. So that gives most of us the additional options of shrimp, muscles, clams, prawns, lobsters, crabs, and octopus. We have to avoid bison (if we're sensitive to beef), because these days, virtually all Bison have DNA from domestic cattle, due to crossbreeding, over the decades.

Safe carbohydrate selections.

The safest vegetable options for most of us are carrots, squash, green beans, Brussels sprouts, kohlrabi, rutabagas, turnips, parsnips, sweet potatoes, yams, cassava, broccoli, cabbage, and cauliflower. Note that the serving size may need to be limited, due to the high fiber content of most of these vegetables. And please note that vegetables such as broccoli and cabbage, especially, typically cause the generation of gas, so those of us who are having trouble with bloating, and eliminating gas, may want to avoid them and other cruciferous vegetables, at least during our recovery journey.

We should avoid commercially processed foods.

At least during our recovery period, we should avoid commercially processed foods, if possible. We need to especially avoid any commercially processed foods that contain more than five ingredients, even if those ingredients are believed to be safe. Gluten-free bread, for example, and most baked products in general, are notorious for causing MC patients to react, despite the fact that all of their ingredients may appear to be safe. Apparently the combination of those ingredients creates digestive problems for many of us. After we've been in remission for a while, and our intestines have had some time to heal, we can test such products, one at a time, for three days, before adding them to our diet.

Many MC patients have trouble selecting foods for breakfast.

If we're sensitive to most conventional breakfast foods, then our breakfasts will tend to look a lot like our other meals, and may consist of warmed-up leftovers from the previous day's meals. We need to be willing to think out-of-the-box, whenever necessary, because sometimes we have to be creative, when our choices are severely limited by food sensitivities. There's no reason why breakfasts have to consist of conventional breakfast foods. They can include virtually any foods that are safe to eat.

Early on, at least during recovery, we should resist the urge to eat commercially processed breakfast cereals, even when their label indicates that they should be safe. Although many are certified to be gluten-free, casein free, soy free, etc., most of them contain too many ingredients, and either one or more of those ingredients, or the combination, can cause us to react, while our immune system is still hypersensitive. And most of them contain preservatives and other additives that may be tolerable after we've been in remission for a while, but while our intestines are still inflamed, and we're trying to reach remission, they're best avoided. As was discussed in the chapter titled Vitamins, Minerals and Methylation Issues, many cereals use some form of vitamin E as a preservative, and the ingredient is derived from soy.

EnteroLab test results may offer additional options.

Those of us who are fortunate enough to not be sensitive to pork, or chicken eggs, have a number of additional breakfast options. If bacon causes problems (and we're not sensitive to pork), we can try uncured bacon. It won't stay fresh nearly as long as cured bacon, but it doesn't contain any of the chemicals normally used in the curing process, in the event those chemicals might cause digestive problems.

Most of us are not sensitive to white potatoes, so hash browns may be a breakfast option. And for those of us not sensitive to corn, grits are a breakfast option.

Minimize reflux risks.

Because acid reflux and GERD are common problems for many MC patients, we may need to be careful not to eat anything within three or four hours of bedtime, especially foods or drinks that promote reflux, such as alcohol (especially red wine), coffee, tea, or soda, chocolate, spicy foods such as black pepper, garlic, or onions, citrus fruits or citrus juice, peppermint, or tomatoes or anything else that we've found may cause us to have reflux problems.

We need to minimize fiber, sugar, and spicy seasonings.

While selecting a recovery diet, we should always be aware that we need to minimize fiber, sugar, and spicy foods. We'll be able to increase the amounts of those foods after we've been in remission for a while, and our digestive system has had some time to heal, but we need to minimize these items in our recovery diet in order to hasten recovery, and minimize the risk that the diet we choose may not bring remission.

We also need to remember to limit our food selections to only a few, bland, safe foods, because this will not only help to ensure that the recovery diet we've selected will reliably bring remission, but it will also shorten the amount of time required to reach remission.

As pointed out in chapter 4, our food is our medicine, so it's important for us to choose the proper "medicine", and it's even more important to not choose any "medicine"that might cause adverse side effects that might prevent us from reaching remission.

Summary

When choosing foods for a recovery diet, ideally, we should choose one to three safe proteins, and one to three safe vegetables, from the lists below. Except in rare cases, these foods are usually safe for most of us. Significant amounts of protein are necessary for healing, so we need to make sure that our diet contains adequate protein. Adequate protein and fat in the diet are essential for good health, but carbohydrates are optional, not essential.

Recovery can be accomplished eating only meat, because meat contains all the essential amino acids that our body needs for good health. But if we choose to go this route, we need to select a fatty meat, or at least make sure that we're ingesting enough fat, so that we avoid the risk of developing the syndrome known as protein poisoning.

We should make sure that we avoid any foods that we were allergic to, or were otherwise sensitive to, before we developed MC. And obviously, if we know that we've become sensitive to any of these foods, since the development of MC, we should continue to avoid them.

Safe Proteins

- turkey
- quail
- duck
- goose
- emu
- lamb
- cabrito (goat)
- venison
- antelope
- rabbit
- shrimp
- muscles
- clams
- prawns
- lobsters
- crabs
- octopus

Safe vegetables

- carrots
- squash
- green beans
- Brussels sprouts
- kohlrabi
- rutabagas
- turnips
- parsnips
- sweet potatoes
- yams
- cassava
- broccoli
- cabbage
- cauliflower

Chapter 7

After Reaching Remission

After remission is achieved, it's best to allow at least a few weeks of healing, before attempting to add foods back into our diet. We need to listen to our body. It will tell us when it's ready. If we feel "bright-eyed and bushy tailed" every morning, then we're probably ready to try to add some foods. On the other hand, if our bowel movements don't seem to be consistently normal, or we feel apprehensive about adding new foods, we probably need to allow more healing time, before trying any new foods. Rushing things can cause a relapse, in some cases.

When we feel that we're ready to begin adding foods back into our diet, we should start by selecting a food that we believe will be safe. We shouldn't, for example, begin by trying to add gluten back into our diet, because gluten will be permanently off-limits, for the rest of our life.

We shouldn't try to add foods that we know are unsafe.

If we have EnteroLab test results showing that we're sensitive to casein or soy, those will probably be permanent sensitivities. A few MC patients who test positive to chicken egg sensitivity, are able to add chicken eggs back into their diet as ingredients in baked goods, for example, but not every one of us is able to do that. Some of us are able to safely eat duck eggs. But again, that doesn't apply to all of us.

Other foods may or may not be safe options.

Other than the big four food sensitivities (gluten, casein, soy, and chicken eggs), the other foods for which EnteroLab has shown positive test results may or may not continue to cause digestive problems. Many of them may eventually be safe food choices for some of us, as we continue to heal, and our immune system slowly reduces its excess sensitivity level. But we need to carefully test these foods (always testing only one food at a time), before adding them back into our diet, and before to even try to add foods, we need to allow adequate healing time, to give our immune system time to settle down.

Those of us who recovered by following an elimination diet, may need to test additional foods.

If we don't have EnteroLab test results showing that we're sensitive to casein or soy, then we should be able to test those foods, one at a time, starting with a small amount and increasing the serving size each day, for three days. If we have a reaction, we should stop eating that food immediately, but if we can eat it for three days without any reaction, then the food is probably safe to add back into our diet, and we can go on to test another food.

If we have a reaction while testing new foods, we need to stop testing foods for a week or two, to give our digestive system time to settle down and stabilize again. After things appear to be back to normal for a few days, we can begin testing new foods again.

We need to go slowly when increasing our fiber and sugar consumption.

Our ability to digest normal amounts of fiber and sugar will slowly improve as our intestines heal. But remember, 2 to 5 years of healing are required for the lining of the intestines to completely heal (return to normal cellular histology), for most adults. That means that most of us may not be able to eat raw salads early on, but after we've been in remission for a while, we may become able to eat small amounts of raw vegetables, and as our digestive system continues to heal, we should eventually be able to eat normal size raw salads.

We should always be cautious about eating out.

Remember the relatively high contamination risks discussed in previous chapters, and whenever important events arise, at which we might decide to eat a meal, it may be helpful to take one of the commercial products designed to assist with the digestion of gluten. These products are not a guarantee against a possible reaction, but they should help to minimize the symptoms, if a reaction does occur. Some of the products in current development and testing, which may soon receive FDA approval, will probably work much better than most of the older products already on the market, that do not have FDA approval.

We need to be cautious, so that we don't allow a reaction to turn into a relapse.

Normally, a reaction against an accidental exposure to gluten, or some other food sensitivity, will end in a day or two. If it doesn't, we need to carefully analyze everything in our diet, looking for a source of cross-contamination. If we're using any commercially processed foods, we should look extra carefully at the labels, in case the manufacturers have changed ingredients.

Flares can be very difficult to resolve.

If we can't track down the problem, we need to stop eating out, stop eating commercially processed foods, and go back to the simple, basic diet that we used to attain remission initially. If the flare was caused by stress, we will probably have to resolve the cause of the stress, before we'll be able to regain remission. If we had to use budesonide to reach remission the last time we were reacting, then we may have to use budesonide again.

If we do have to use budesonide, we need to start the treatment with the full 9 mg per day dose, taken all at once, first thing in the morning, because that maximizes the effectiveness of all corticosteroids. Taking a smaller dose might work, eventually, but in most cases, it either will not work, or it will take a long time to gain control of the inflammation, and stop the reaction. If we do use budesonide, we should be sure to taper the dose very, very slowly, when weaning off the drug.

Refractive symptoms may be due to an infection.

We should always be aware that MC patients are still subject to all of the digestive system diseases and infections that everyone else in the general population has to deal with, occasionally. If a flare does not respond to treatment, and especially if there is blood in our stool, we should suspect an infection.

In such a situations, we'll need to visit our doctor (our primary care doctor should be able to handle this), and request a stool culture to check for an infection caused by parasites, or pathogenic bacteria. Sometimes, especially if the infection is due to certain issues such as C. diff, the culture may have to be repeated a time or two in order to detect and identify the bacteria causing the infection

Our diet should allow us to control our microscopic colitis symptoms indefinitely.

Using the information in this book, we should be able to keep the symptoms of the disease under control for the rest of our life. In some cases, additional food sensitivities may develop later, and if that happens, we have to fine-tune our diet to allow for any additional food sensitivities. But normally, additional food sensitivities don't develop.

Whenever any dietary MC issues arise, by referring to the guidelines in this book, we should be able to resolve the problem. Life is good, when microscopic colitis is kept under control.

The Microscopic Colitis Diet Book

Summary

We should always test any new foods before adding them into our diet. And we should always listen to our body, especially when trying to add new foods into our diet. Some food sensitivities, such as gluten, casein, and soy, are permanent, while others may eventually resolve as our digestive system heals, and our immune system sensitivity settles back down to normal.

We have to allow some time for our digestive system to heal, before adding certain new foods back into our diet, and before significantly increasing our fiber and sugar intake. We should always be aware of the relatively high risk of cross-contamination in most restaurant meals, especially before our digestive system has had a year or two of healing. Flares happen, and when they do, it behooves us to resolve them as quickly as possible, because if they continue to develop, they can be very difficult to resolve. And we have to remember that we're subject to the same digestive system issues that almost everyone in the general population has to deal with occasionally.

The tools needed to keep this disease under control by using proper dietary management are discussed in detail in this book. Most of us are able to keep our disease under control for the rest of our life, by carefully following these guidelines.

About the Author

Wayne Persky

Wayne Persky was born, grew up, and currently lives in Central Texas. He is a graduate of the University of Texas at Austin, College of Engineering, with postgraduate studies in mechanical engineering, mathematics, and computer science. He has teaching experience in engineering, and business experience in farming, grain processing, and agribusiness.

In 2005, he founded, and continues to administrate an online microscopic colitis discussion and support forum. In 2015 he founded the Microscopic Colitis Foundation, and he continues to serve as it's president and as a contributing author to the Foundation's Newsletter.

He has spent over 20 years researching food sensitivities, and vitamin and mineral deficiencies, and how they effect our health. Currently, he continues to research published medical journals, and write about health issues that the medical community fails to adequately address.

Contact Details:

Wayne Persky can be contacted at:

The Microscopic Colitis Diet Book

Persky Farms
19242 Darrs Creek Rd
Bartlett, TX 76511
USA

Tel: 1(254)718-1125
Tel: 1(254)527-3682

Email: pfarms@perskyfarms.com
Email: wayne@microscopiccolitisfoundation.org
Email: wayne@waynepersky.com

For information and support regarding microscopic colitis, visit:

https://www.microscopiccolitisfoundation.org/
To view or participate in the Microscopic Colitis Discussion and Support Forum, go to:

https://www.perskyfarms.com/phpBB/index.php

1   Hollon, J., Puppa, E. L., Greenwald, B., Goldberg, E., Guerrerio, A., & Fasano, A. (2015). Effect of gliadin on permeability of intestinal biopsy explants from celiac disease patients and patients with non-celiac gluten sensitivity. Nutrients, 7(3), 1565–1576. Retrieved from https://pubmed.ncbi.nlm.nih.gov/25734566/

2   Long, M. (2022, March 16). Review highlights unmet need for more effective therapies in Crohn's. Retrieved from https://www.medpagetoday.com/reading-room/aga/inflammatorydisease/97683

3   Münch, A., Bohr, J., Miehlke, S., Benoni, C., Olesen, M., Öst, Å., Strandberg, L., . . . Ström, M. (2016). Low-dose budesonide for maintenance of clinical remission in collagenous colitis: a randomised, placebo-controlled, 12-month trial. *Gut*, 65(1),47–56. Retrieved from https://gut.bmj.com/content/65/1/47

4   Laffin, M., Fedorak, R., Zalasky, A., Park, H.,Gill, A., Agrawal, A., & Madsen, K. (2019). A high-sugar diet rapidly enhances susceptibility to colitis via depletion of luminal short-chain fatty acids in mice. Scientific Reports 9, 12294. Retrieved from https://www.na-ture.com/articles/s41598-019-48749-2

5   Tye-Din, J. A., Stewart, J. A., Dromey, J. A., Beissbarth, T., van Heel, D. A., Tatham, A. . . . Anderson, R. P. (2010). Comprehensive, Quantitative Mapping of T Cell Epitopes in Gluten in Celiac Disease. *Science Translational Medicine*, 2(41), p41–51. Retrieved from

https://www.science.org/doi/10.1126/scitranslmed.3001
012?url_ver=Z39.88-2003&rfr_id=ori%3Arid%3Across-
ref.org&rfr_dat=cr_pub++0pubmed&

6   Kasarda, D. D. (n.d). Grains in Relation to Celiac
(Coeliac) Disease. *USDA*. Retrieved from
https://wheat.pw.usda.gov/ggpages/topics/celiac.html

7   Scaglione, F., and Panzavolta, G. (2014). Folate, folic
acid and 5-methyltetrahydrofolate are not the same
thing. Xenobiotica, 44(5),490–488, Retrieved from
https://pubmed.ncbi.nlm.nih.gov/24494987/

8   Thorne. (n.d.). What is Methylation and Why Should
You Care About it. Retrieved from
https://www.thorne.com/take-5-daily/article/what-is-
methylation-and-why-should-you-care-about-it

9   Narula, N., Cooray, M., Anglin, R., Muqtadir, Z.,
Narula, A., & Marshall, J. K. (2017). *Digestive Diseases
and Sciences*, (62), 448–455. Retrieved from
https://link.springer.com/article/10.1007%2Fs10620-
016-4396-7

10 Raftery, T., and O'Sullivan, M. (2015). Optimal vitamin
D levels in Crohn's disease: a review. *Proceedings of the
Nutrition Society*, (24)1, 56–66. Retrieved from
https://www.cambridge.org/core/journals/proceed-
ings-of-the-nutrition-society/article/optimal-vitamin-d-
levels-in-crohns-disease-a-
review/E041A64165B65124937A5652A55E62EE

11 Taub, P. R., Manson, J-A. E., & Holick, M. F. (2021, December 01). Beyond Bone Health: Does Vitamin D Have a Role in Cancer, CVD, and COVID? [Web log message] Retrieved from https://www.medscape.com/viewarticle/959893? uac=95382HN&faf=1&sso=true&impID=3841253&src= mkm_covid_update_211201_MSCPEDIT

12 Trinity College Dublin. (2021, December 14). Vitamin B12 deficiency increases risk of depression. *Psychology & Psychiatry*, Retrieved from https://medicalx-press.com/news/2021-12-vitamin-b12-deficiency-de-pression.html

13 Office of Dietary Supplements. (n.d.). Vitamin E. Retrieved from https://ods.od.nih.gov/factsheets/Vita-minE-HealthProfessional/

14 Jiang, Q., Christen, S., Shigenaga, M. K., & Ames, B. N. (2001). γ-Tocopherol, the major form of vitamin E in the US diet, deserves more attention. *The American Journal of Clinical Nutrition*, 74(6), 714–722. Retrieved from https://academic.oup.com/ajcn/article/74/6/714/4737392

Printed in the USA
CPSIA information can be obtained
at www.ICGtesting.com
LVHW010721190224
772164LV00002B/217